Herbal Medicine Collection:
60 DIY Herbal Remedies for Health & Healing

20 Herbs and Herbal Mixes to Healthy Living and Healing

Introduction: The Best Things Come from Scratch!

About as far back as conscious, human recollection goes, herbs from man's natural environment have been used for medicinal purposes. They were used in India over 5000 years ago in the form of Ayurvedic Medicine. And in ancient Greece, for a physician named Aristotle, the power of flowers, fruits, seeds and roots, was just what the doctor ordered.

Herbal medicine was the standard form of treatment for much of the world for centuries. In the past when someone was sick they would pay a visit to their local herbal expert who would find just the right ingredient to help them. A sorely missed ingredient for most of us in modern life, since in much of the prepackaged and mass produced modern world, we are hard pressed to even find herbs in the food we eat, let alone are medicine. But as this book bears testament—things are starting to change!

And herbal therapies are starting to make a major come back. And one of the most popular herbal therapies to make some headway is that of Aromatherapy. With its roots firmly affixed to the incense burners of the ancient world, this herbal practice has us purposefully inhaling the fragrance of specific herbs in order to create a desired reaction in our body. A powerful treatment that has now sprung up as special Aromatherapy clinics attached to many major hospitals.

In recent years the use of taking the essential oils from medicinal herbs and using them in specifically targeted massage therapy has also become in vogue. We will discuss both of these practices and many more methods further in this book. For right now I just want to captivate your imagination with the possibilities and ignite your awareness of the impact that these powerful medicinal herbs can have on your life.

Sometimes known as holistic medicine, medicinal herbs are used to treat the whole body. This holistic approach is something that modern medicine often lacks. Because often enough, when we turn to pharmaceuticals we find ourselves just masking chronic symptoms, whereas many herbal medicines are able to target the actual deficiency itself, which is the source of the problem. Showing once again that, most of our aches and pains are simply our body crying out for something that it lacks.

Because when you break it all down, just as the Christian/Hebrew bible and many other ancient religious traditions remind us; we came from the dust of the Earth. We truly are part and parcel to this planet, and all of the molecules, all of the proteins, amino acids and other trace elements in our body can be found strewn all over the Earth. So if this is from whence we came, and we find that our body is lacking something, all we have to do is look to the Earth to find it. We don't need to replicate and synthesize chemicals in a pharmacy; all we have to do is look to nature and the medicines that it naturally provides. Because the best things truly do come from scratch!

Chapter 1: Aromatherapy; A Nose above the Rest!

The human nose is an intricate piece of sensory machinery, we may not be aware of the complexities involved in smelling a cup of coffee, but that doesn't mean that they are not there. Called the "Chemosensory System" the nose is part of a joint apparatus that works to use the senses of taste and smell in order to help us interpret our environment.

For thousands of years our sense of smell has served to help us find a meal, tell us of potential threats, and through pheromones that trigger powerful chemosensory responses, has even played a role in determining our mates. We may take it for granted and not realize how influential are noses are, but just try to go a few days without it and you will quickly realize what you are missing.

Our noses work hard to interpret our environment, constantly labeling and cataloging a vast multitude of chemical molecules that we inhale every time we breathe in the air. In an instant our nose is able to pick up the distinct chemical trace element of a campfire and then send it to our brain which instantly relates to us our fond memories of when we used to go camping with our Uncle Bernie.

Every time we smell a specific "smell" it is due to the fact that an odor molecule has bonded to one of the millions of "olfactory receptors" in our nasal cavity whose job is to interpret what those odor molecules are. Telling us whether something is bitter, salty, sweet, or one of a million variations in between. These incredibly complex interchanges happen in an instant—and faster than you can say, "This stinks!"—your nose is way ahead of you relaying that information!

As you can see, the nose is on the front line of our senses and working as a great interpreter of what is good for us, and what is not so good for us in the chemical makeup of our world. The nose also works as a natural gateway when it comes to the field of herbal medicine. It was also the original "gateway drug" in ancient religious practice in which incense was a common feature of inducing more mindful states for ceremonies and to relieve the stress of participants.

Frankincense

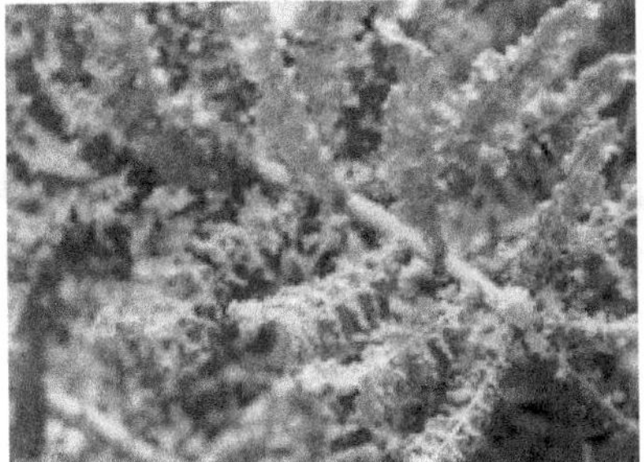

Powerful herbs were burned by the boatload in order to set the mood of the faithful. Smelling powerful incense was always a powerful part of religious service, making medicinal herbs a highly prized possession. And one of the most famous of these herbs is that of "Frankincense". Who could forget this wonder drug of the ancients? This was a medicinal herb that was so spectacular that it even made a cameo in the first Christmas story. Does anyone remember the three Magi who carried their Frankincense and Myrrh all the way from Persia?

In ancient times this stuff was of such high value that it was sometimes doled out as its own kind of currency. Frankincense was known to be able to alter the chemistry of the brain just by inhaling its fragrance. When the ancients were feeling a bit down in the doldrums they would just burn incense laced with Frankincense for an all natural herbal pick-me-up. And besides the elevation of mood it was discovered to have great affect on treating many kinds of inflammation.

It was quite a common practice for the local apothecary of yesteryear to either massage a bit of Frankincense into their patient's aching joints, or to have them just take a deep breath of their burning Frankincense cauldrons. Because just the smell of Frankincense alone can kick start a powerful chemical reaction in the body that cleanses it from impurities and boosts the immune system.

In modern day Ayurvedic circles Frankincense has even been known to fight cancer. Studies have shown that the application of Frankincense can reduce the onset or even reverse the incidence of Basil Cell Carcinoma (Skin Cancer), demonstrating exactly why this medicinal herb continues to be such a valuable commodity to this very day. Just by taking a breath of fresh air we can revitalize our entire system.

This is the basic premise that aromatherapy has been based on. But besides incense, one of the other traditional ways to take in the fragrance of medicinal herbs is to make an old fashioned poultice. A poultice is a distribution method of directly applying herbs to the skin, often around the neck and shoulders, so that the aroma of the herbs can be directly inhaled over a long period of time.

Poultices usually consist of dried out plant material rather than liquid and are crushed or mashed together and boiled with water before their application in order to make the ingredients more malleable so they can be easily pasted onto the skin. The poultice is often held onto the chest or neck area as a compress, fixed in place with heavy gauze.

Chamomile

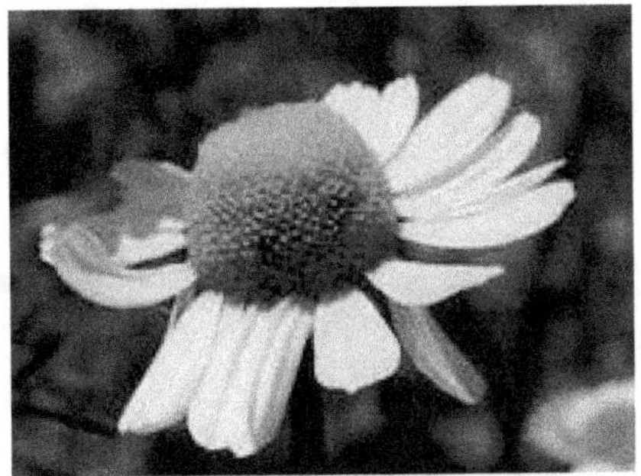

The herb Chamomile which is most famously known for its properties in tea also doubles as a great poultice. The crushed petals of the Chamomile flower compressed over a bruise or area of severe inflammation can bring immediate relief through this powerful poultice. The Chamomile poultice is also effective when placed on the jaw to relieve toothaches or around the ear to relieve a bad earache. But as mentioned you don't have to wear a poultice to get the effects of Chamomile.

Because a good strong blend of Chamomile tea can do wonders to alleviate muscle aches, as well as improve symptoms of anxiety and depression. And along with relaxing our nerves, breathing in the aroma of Chamomile has also been shown to relax our blood vessels, helping us to keep our blood pressure under control.

In order to get a good whiff of tea variety Chamomile make yourself a steaming hot mug and pour the tea into the mug hot. And before you even drink it, just put your face close and cup your hands around the mug and your nose, letting yourself breathe in deep the aroma of your tea. You can also just pull up a chair to your tea kettle and simply sit by the stove breathing in the steady aroma steaming out of your tea pot. Either way the effect is the same.

Bergamot

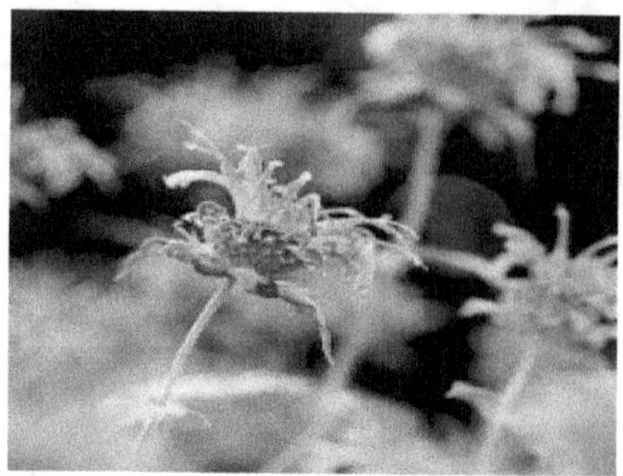

Very similar to the effects of Chamomile, is that of Bergamot, another relaxation inducing herb that can be used in either incense, a poultice wrap or in a great tasting cup of tea. Along with aiding relaxation, Bergamot has some other additional medicinal properties completely unique to this herb. With one of them being its amazing propensity to enable the body to completely neutralize the effects of fevers. Bergamot also works as a powerful disinfectant and antioxidant.

Due to its notable healing properties with the skin this herbal remedy is often taken with a bath either by placing a few drops of Bergamot essential oil (we will discuss essential oils further in the next chapter) or by specially manufactured soaps that have the Bergamot baked right in. Either way, with all of these powerful aromatic options, you will be head and shoulders (and head and nose) above the rest!

Chapter 2: Healing Through Essential Oils

Essential Oils are basically a refined gathering of plant based matter in liquid form. Inside this broad grouping of gathered plant material, we can break Essential Oils down into 8 main categories. They are; floral, citrus, herbaceous, spicy, resinous, earthy, and camphoraceous. All of these categories of Essential Oils are known to serve different purposes. But probably the most widely used however, are those that are derived from the floral family of essential oils.

Rose

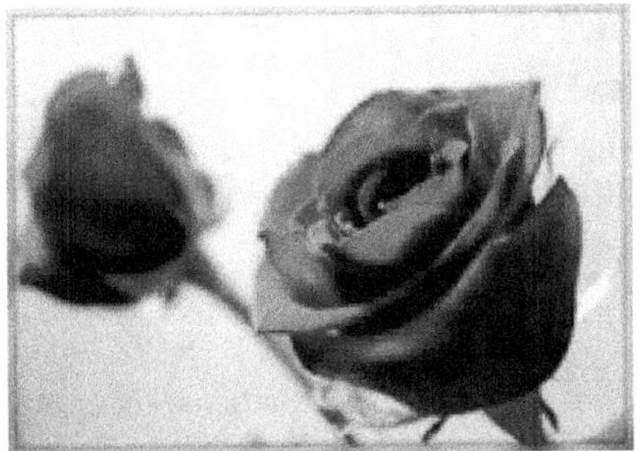

You don't have to look much farther than the expression, "It's time to stop and smell the roses." To realize just how widespread our attachment to floral fauna is. Roses in particular have been known to have many positive medicinal effects on the human body. For example, the petals from a rose when ground into essential oil have been known to be able to treat insomnia, stress, and depression. It has also been widely reported to be able to work as an anti-viral agent that helps boost the immune system.

Geranium

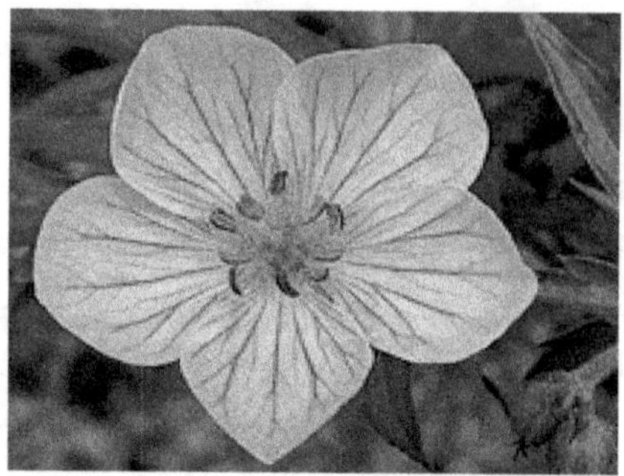

But as good as the rose is, it is also a costly herbal remedy, so much so, that many have opted to use its closest cousin instead. Because the oil derived from the Geranium is known to be nearly identical to oil derived from roses. Its benefits are also very similar, like roses the Geranium is known to have an immediate stress relieving quality when used in aromatherapy or when the oil is massaged into the skin.

Just like the roses, this essential oil also has powerful anti-viral and immune system boosting properties. Geranium oil also works extraordinarily well as a treatment for some of the side effects that women experience during their menstrual cycle as well as helping to alleviate the symptoms of menopause. Another reason that many women swear by this essential oil is also due to its widely known ability to reduce stretch marks which of course is a welcome relief after pregnancy.

But whether it is used for men or women, the compounds found in Geranium essential oil have been known to be able to completely balance out our hormones and help us function on a more even keel. Germanium as a relaxing agent helps to make our muscles contract, it aids our blood vessels in their constriction, and even works to loosen up digestive systems that are plagued with indigestion.

The other interesting thing about Geranium oil is that it is what we call in the world of aromatherapy, a "circulatory oil". This means that rather than releasing the chemical compounds directly upon exhalation—as is the case with other fragrances—the inhalation of Geranium sticks with us and instead of leaving when we breathe out, it goes straight to our blood where it continues to circulate in the body.

But even though we don't exhale the molecules out, they do have to leave the body eventually, and it is the method in which Geranium leaves us that creates another pleasant side effect. Geranium essential oil can only leave us when it is sweated out of the skin. Turning the user of this substance into a living, breathing air freshener, emitting the attractive scent of Geranium just from perspiring! This can have many medicinal uses for someone if they suffer from excessive body odor and it has been known to work as a treatment due to its great deodorizing effects.

Lotus

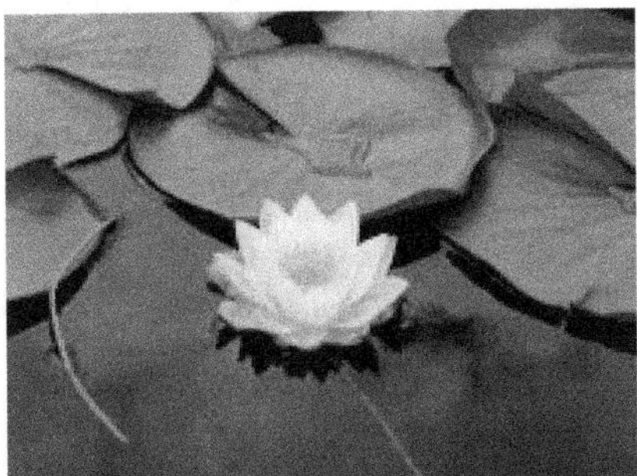

But probably one of the most celebrated oils to ever be extracted from a medicinal herb is that of Lotus oil. Known in the Eastern Hemisphere for thousands of years, the lotus blossom has been the stuff of legend. Along with countless Indian Yogi's down through the centuries, it is said that Buddha himself had prescribed this medicinal herb to his followers, making this medicinal herb a hallmark of two major religions.

But it is the essential oil extracted from this plant that can really create some mind blowing effects. Because just a little bit of lotus oil opens up the lungs and induces a feeling of calm. It would seem to be no coincidence then that the "lotus position" that has become so synonymous with Buddhism and meditation is associated with this flower. The lotus and its oil can have a major impact on our feelings of well being.

Jasmine

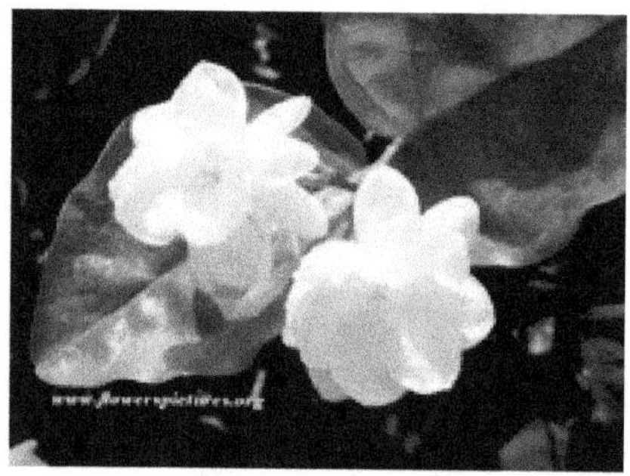

Right next to the effects of the oil from the Lotus, Jasmine essential oil is also a powerful medicinal herb in its own right. Coming from a flower that carries the moniker of "King of Flowers" the scent of Jasmine is unmistakable. I can testify about this from my own personal experience because years ago my senses were frequently inundated with this lovely sent in the most unlikely of places.

When I was still in college I used to do payroll for a truck company and right outside the door to our office someone had planted a ton of these Jasmine flowers and every spring when the flowers bloomed, we were all overwhelmed with their powerful scent. And whoever walked in the door when these flowers were nearby seemed to instantly perk up to their fragrance.

Even the big burly truck drivers who were on layover at our facility seemed to become rather pleasant and tranquil with this aroma around. Showing that even the toughest and gruffest of truck drivers need to take the time to smell the roses! Yet another example of just how soothing and medicinal the essential oils from these herbs can be; providing a bit of healing for us all.

Chapter 3: The Herbal Medicine Cabinet

Most of the time we are always hearing about the "latest" advances in medicine and high tech methods to treat illnesses. But what about some of the low tech options such as medicinal herbs that have been with us for thousands of years?

Because no matter what you may be up against, whatever sickness or ailment that you may be facing the immense bounty of nature and its medicinal herbs is bound to have the solution you are looking for. So let's stock up our low tech medicine cabinet on some of the most important medicinal herbs for daily health, as well as emergencies.

Echinacea

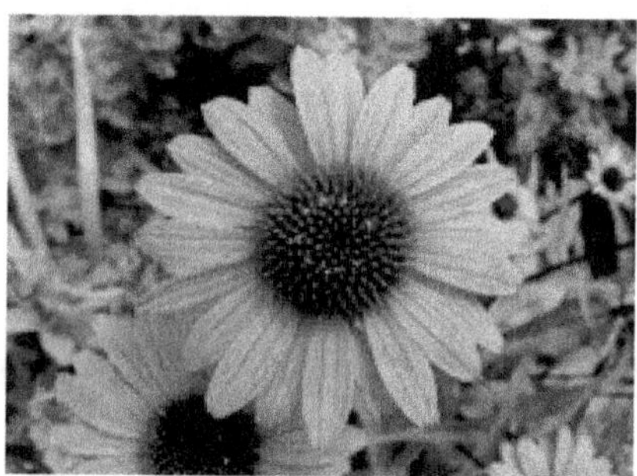

The first addition to our herbal medicine cabinet has been used by Native Americans for years for its anti-viral and anti-biotic properties. Echinacea is a potent herb and when ground into powder or the oil is extracted it is a powerful fighting agent against germs, viruses, bacteria, and even warts! So be sure to stock your herbal medicine cabinet with this precious resource.

Aloe Vera

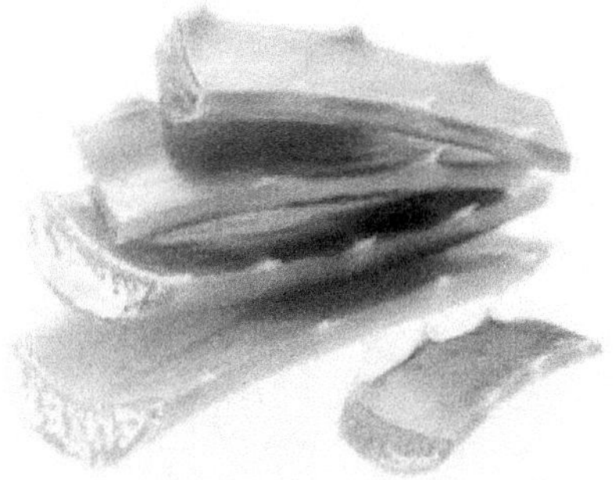

Growing up in Florida, as a child I learned from first hand experience that if you live in an environment with a lot of sunshine then Aloe Vera can be your best friend. Aloe Vera has been used to treat sunburns for a long time and is fast becoming standard fare even in burn units at hospitals. So if you are out in the sun and wind up with a bad burn it could help you out quite a bit if you have some of this stuff on hand.

Nowadays this Aloe Vera is fairly ubiquitous and you can find it at just about any CVS or Walgreens drugstore, but you don't have to buy it, because you can always just make your own. I'm a big fan of DIY and truly believe in the mantra that if you can do it yourself; then you might as well do it!

In order to make your own Aloe Vera you will need a leaf from the Aloe Vera Plant, the leaves of this plant are naturally full of the very same gel that you would buy at the drug store. So just take a leaf off this plant and either break it or cut it with a knife or scissors and squeeze the gel out into a small bowl.

After you've squeezed the gel into your bowl you can go ahead and scoop it out with a spoon or your fingers and apply it directly to your skin. Or if you would like to save it for later simply cover the bowl and put it in a cool and dry place such as a cabinet or possibly a first aid kit.

Catnip

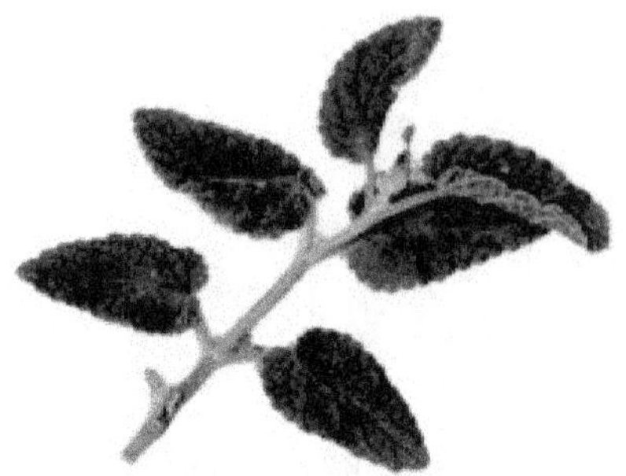

Our next recommendation for your low tech medicine cabinet is probably going to come as a bit of a surprise (for you and your cat) because as it turns out, catnip has many medicinal properties beyond making your feline friends go berserk. Catnip when used properly (for humans) is a natural cure for insomnia. Ground up leaves from the Catnip plant can be used to make medicinal teas that help sooth and relax those who drink them..

This same relaxing effect is also known to relax the digestive system, so if you are having stomach issues drinking a relaxing blend of catnip tea may be just the thing to put your troubled stomach at ease. It's also been well documented in its ability to help relieve headaches, so whether you are having trouble with your nerves, your sleep, your stomach or just have a nasty migraine, a medicinal blend of this catnip herb just might help you out.

Mistletoe

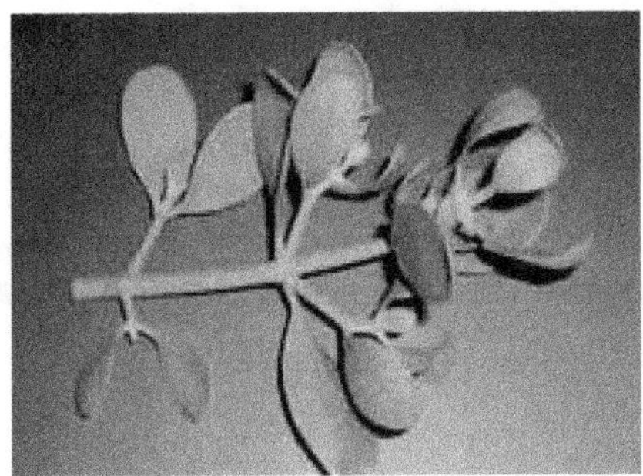

Another medicinal herb you may be surprised to find as a must have in your Herbal Medicine Cabinet is that of the most notorious hanger-on the holiday season has ever known; the Mistletoe. Yes, yes, I know you are probably rolling your eyes as you fight to keep "Ho, Ho, the Mistletoe!" from becoming stuck in your head, but please hear me out. Because this thing has a medicinal worth that goes far beyond holiday smooching.

For a plant that has such loving connotations, the Mistletoe's origins are actually that of a parasite. Normally found attached to Oak and Hawthorn trees, the Mistletoe receives its nourishment by leeching onto other plants. The great thing the Mistletoe does when it attaches itself to the nervous system of humans however, is that it has been found to be a wonderful anti-spasmodic agent that works well in treating convulsive nervous disorders such as epilepsy.

The leaves of this plant have been valued for quite a long time as a nervine and antispasmodic herbal medicine. In the past Mistletoe leaves have even been used to treat hysteria. Teas from Mistletoe leaves have also been known to help slow down a rapid heart rate, relieve high blood pressure, and soothe aching bones. But a word of caution however, the berries of this plant are mildly toxic and people have been known to get sick from eating them. The berries of the Mistletoe should be left alone; any medicinal properties of this plant should be derived from the leaves.

__Garlic__

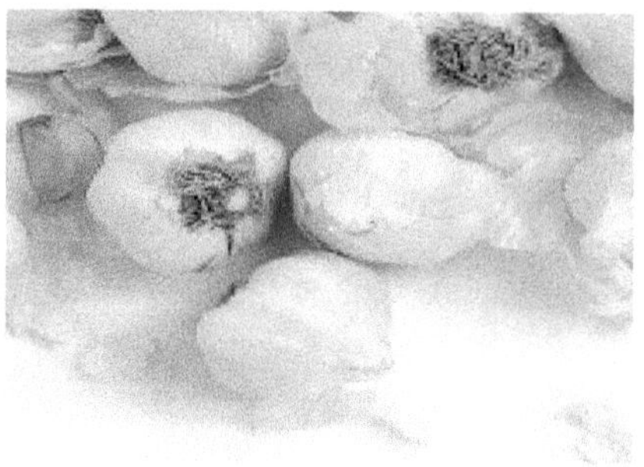

For the next installment in the herbal medicine cabinet we are going to suggest an herbal remedy that can work as an amazing antiseptic and immune booster as well as being rather tasty as a pizza topping. The herb I am talking about is Garlic. Known for its healing properties on the battlefields of the ancient world, crushed cloves of garlic applied directly to cuts and scrapes greatly speeds up the body's ability to heal its wounds.

Garlic is also known to be an incredible immune booster insulating the body well against colds and the flu, making this tasty medicinal herb a definite addition to the herbal medicine cabinet during the cold and flu season. This herb is best in its natural state, so keep a few cloves around that you can grind into powder or boil into your foods.

__Astragalus__

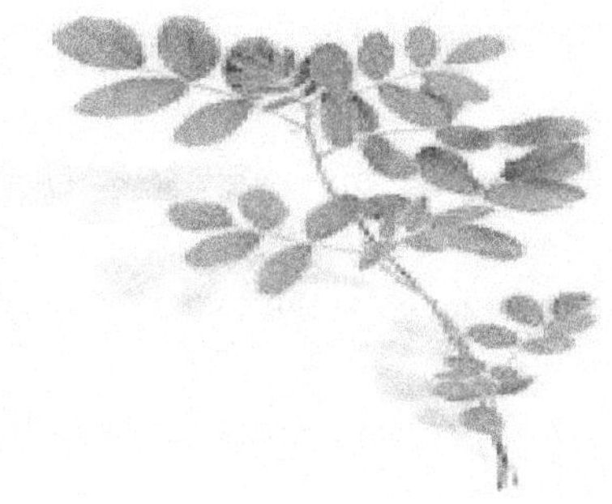

The Chinese herb Astragalus should be another addition to your herbal medicine cabinet. This herb has been used in Chinese medicine for years and is an excellent way to boost the immune system, fight colds, and energize the body. Astragalus is gathered as a root and usually ground into fine powder for use. It can either be applied directly to the skin or boiled in tea.

Dandelion

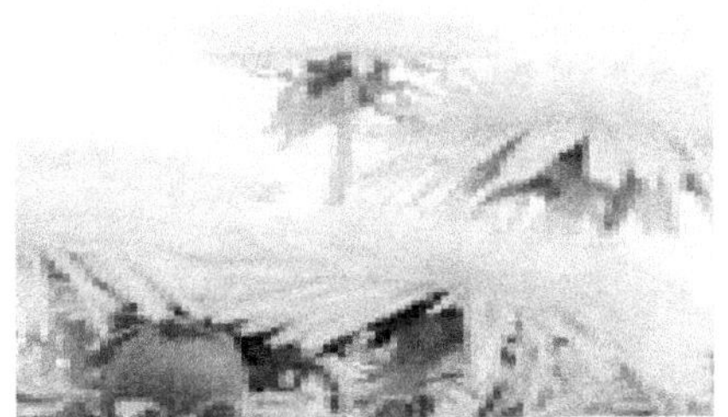

Although this herb is native to Europe it has become quite ubiquitous in North America as well. Known as the "backyard herbal remedy" in a real pinch the Dandelion can be quite useful. Dandelion roots can be drunk as a kind of tonic in teas and even "root" beers. The medicinal benefits of this magical root range from helping to aid indigestion all the way to promoting proper insulin function in diabetics. Providing powerful benefits for your health and making for a great addition to your Herbal Medicine Cabinet.

Chapter 4: Herbal Aids for Weight Loss

With so many people suffering from expanding waist lines, in recent years we are flooded with a never ending litany of dieting fads and gimmicks. Carb restricting regimens such as Atkins and the Paleo diet in particular have become very popular as of late, but the only problem is, once you deviate away from these strict carb reducing regimens the weight comes right back.

The world of herbal medicine when it comes to weight loss has not been immune to criticisms either, as was most famously evidenced from the fallout Dr. Alan Hirsch faced a few years ago over his failed "Sensa" weight loss powder. Do you remember that? Sensa was a supposed aromatherapy based blend of aromatic crystals that people were told to sprinkle over their food to help them lose weight.

The jury still seems to be out on Dr. Hirsch's method, and if it actually worked, but when it comes to whether or not his clients had the right to sue him on false advertising, the jury emphatically agreed in the form of a 26 million dollar lawsuit. But what if we could bypass those mysterious "aromatic crystals" of Sensa and turn to a few proven herbal ingredients to enhance our diet and help to manage our weight the natural way? Look no further than "Rosemary".

Rosemary

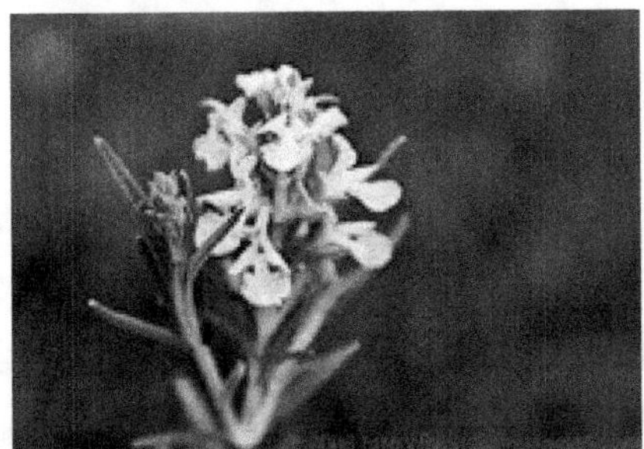

This medicinal herb hails from Asia and has been held in acclaim far and wide for its beneficial properties in regard to regulating weight gain and even eliminating cellulite. When this herb is consumed in a cup of tea it can raise your metabolism helping you to burn fat. Rosemary is also an excellent diuretic and the first weight that this herb will help you lose will undoubtedly be water weight, as this tea directly cleanses your system of excess water and other toxins.

After de-toxing like this, the Rosemary coursing through your system will bring you a new surge of energy and wellness; refreshing you as it cleanses. If you drink this tea for seven days straight your body will be primed, and streamlined with a higher metabolism and completely cleansed of toxins.

Rosemary works to eliminate any previous digestion problems, getting rid of bloating and helping you to break down food faster. As a result you will feel content with your food intake faster, curbing your appetite and keeping you from eating more. Most people lose at least a few pounds after their first weak of exposure to Rosemary and many more claim that this herb has toned their body and eliminated their unsightly cellulite.

Peppermint

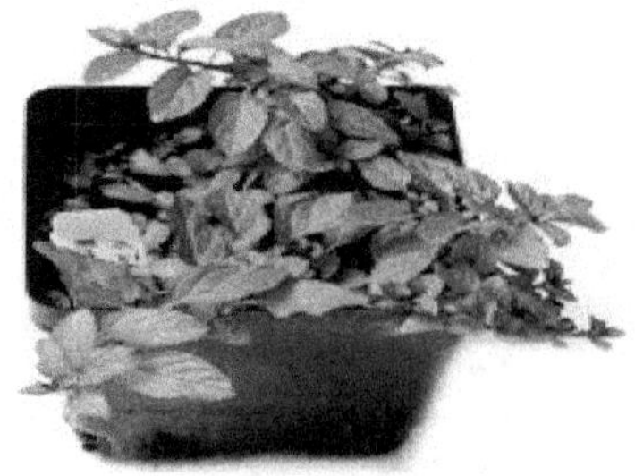

Another good herbal cleanser for the body is peppermint. Peppermint when inhaled and absorbed through the skin can directly influence bile secretion in the digestive tract. An action that helps to suppress appetite and further kick start your metabolism. Peppermint is best burned as incense and inhaled directly or even in a nice warm bath absorbing a diluted amount in your bathwater.

Ginseng

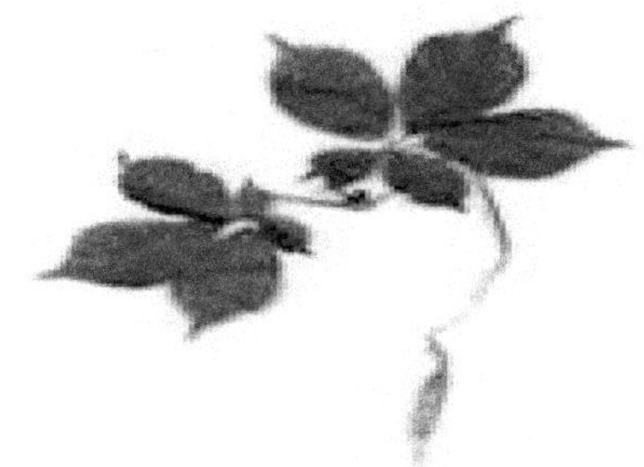

Last but certainly not least in our quest for herbal weight loss is the ancient Chinese herb of Ginseng. The roots from this herb are potent and have been known to boost the metabolism, but much more than this, Ginseng has the uncanny ability to alter the body's cells directly, altering their composition and actually rendering them less capable of storing fat. This herb and all the others mentioned in this chapter are most definitely welcome news for anyone seeking an herbal aid for weight loss.

Chapter 5: Herbs for Health, Beauty, and Cosmetics

Medicinal herbs can be a powerful force of healing in just about every aspect of our lives, beauty and cosmetics is yet another area where these natural remedies can apply. And if you are like 99.9% of the rest of the people on this planet, you probably tend to be a little bit concerned about your hair. Don't worry though because our herbs have us covered in that department as well. Because if you would like to have shiny healthy hair all you need is a few drops of a special little herb called "Sandalwood".

Sandalwood

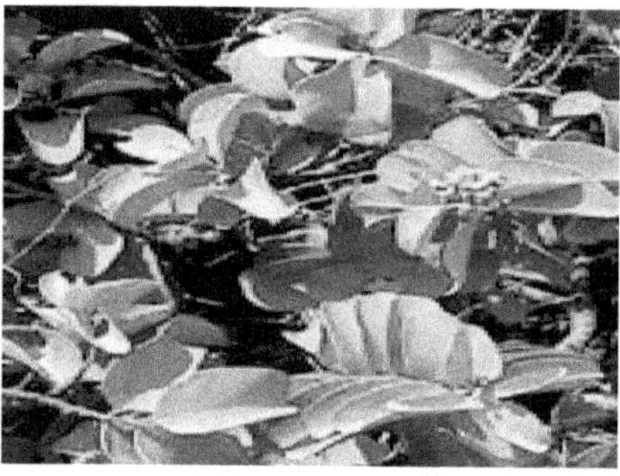

Sandalwood works as a powerful cleansing agent and along with shinier hair, sandalwood does a remarkable job of rejuvenating the skin and enhancing the user's overall complexion. Sandalwood can also work as an active ingredient in relieving the symptoms of Eczema and other skin disorders. Even better for those of us that have already sailed past the age of 30, Sandalwood is known to reduce the appearance of wrinkles. Sandalwood can work its way right under those bags under your eyes, reduce the moisture and make them disappear!

A great homemade mixture for Sandalwood skin cream involves one tablespoon of Sandalwood powder combined with a tablespoon of turmeric in about half a cup of water. Just apply this mixture as a paste to the skin and you will begin to see results right away. Let the paste dry off naturally and you will soon find that your skin has a clear and natural sheen.

Rosewood

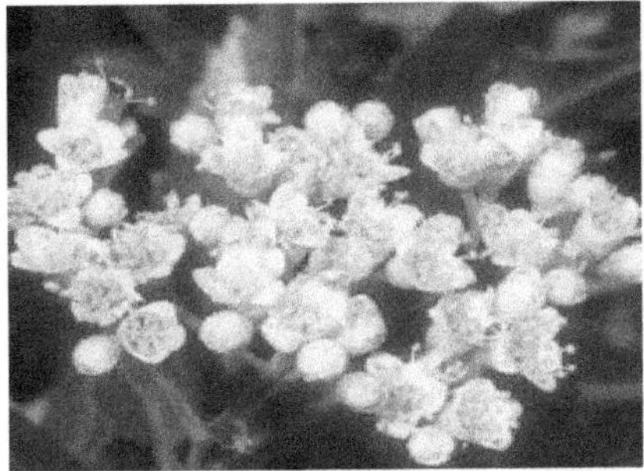

Rosewood is also a great herb for healthy skin and hair, and has been used in soap and shampoo since at least the early 1900's. Rosewood is extracted primarily from trees native to the great rainforests of South America, a fact that has unfortunately led to some pretty bad deforestation. Recent conservation legislation however has fought against this and the extraction of rosewood is highly regulated in order to prevent abuse and unnecessary waste of this precious resource.

Avocado

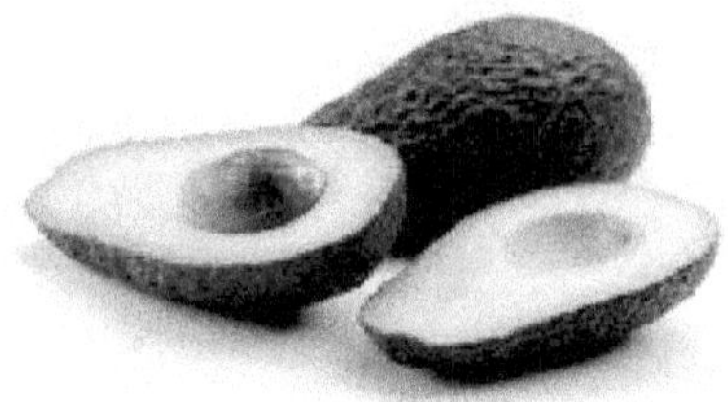

Our next notable mention for cosmetic enhancement you have probably used before to enhance your tacos! I'm talking about Avocados of course! Avocados have long played a role in that familiar face mask that many women (and some men) have ritually went to bed with over the years. It's sometimes remembered more as a running gag in TV sitcoms than as a viable health therapy, but a good Avocado moisturizer mask really can help your skin.

The active ingredient in an Avocado's oil is Vitamin D which works to penetrate and nourish the skin, helping to rejuvenate it and encouraging new tissue growth, allowing the surface level of our epidermal cells to stay younger longer. So if your wife ever scared you in the middle of the night by plastering her face up in so much bright green Avocado oil that you woke up thinking a space alien was in bed with you; don't get mad! Because the benefits of this medicinal treatment, and all of the others mentioned in this chapter, far outweigh the discomfort!

Conclusion: Staying Healthy For Life

In the stress filled world of today, staying healthy can seem like a regular 9 to 5 job. The number one complaint for most of us is that we just don't have time to take care of our health. This is the reason why so many of us today would like to just pop a quick pill to get over whatever is bothering us. But unfortunately there is no quick fix when it comes to our health.

We need to break away from our preconceived and prepackaged notions and reintroduce ourselves to the resources that nature can provide. As we have learned in this book, herbal medicine has been with us for a long time, and it isn't going anywhere anytime soon. Everything we could ever need is right there in front of us, we just have to know how to take it. Once we do, healthy living and healing will not be far behind.

Preppers Survival Medicine:

Introduction

While considering the use of medicinal plants, you have to find out the type of injury you have. Various plants are used for the treatment of multiple scenarios, but you have to select a right plant for your injury. You have to find out either you are bleeding or suffering from inflammation. If there is something oozing or you want something for diarrhea. It is essential to get the advantage of the right plant because a wrong medicinal plant can be an invitation to a new problem. Keep it in mind that you can mix plants together to increase their medicinal properties.

If you are having a bite, you may need a drawing agent to remove any toxic substance and an antihistamine to reduce itching. Make sure to be creative, but stay away from dangerous plants. It can be risky for you to use a poisonous plant. With the help of universal edibility test, you can find out ingestible medicinal plants. For instance, boneset is a peculiar plant and you can identify it with its unique look because its stems look pierce through the middle of the leaves. This plant is really fantastic because it can help you to treat flu and cold. Its taste is awful, but it works really well. You can wrap it around your wound to increase the speed of healing. It can be consumed raw or infuse in a tea.

It is a single example, but there are various plants that are really safe and good for medicinal use. It will be good to learn about potential plants found in the wilderness and you can use them as a medicine. This book offers almost 15 herbs and plants that are safe for you and improve your health. You can use them to save the life of any person. Read this book and learn about these plants and herbal medicines:

Chapter 01: Plants and Herbs that can Save Your Life in the Wilderness

Living out in the wild, you'll run over a wide range of therapeutic plants and restorative herbs that can be utilized for various purposes, the length of you know where to look and how to utilize them. Numerous plants are valuable for sustenance, as well as can be utilized as medication also.

Plants can be utilized to mitigate a wide range of illnesses. Everything from skin rash, joint inflammation, cool, fever, looseness of the bowels, headaches, and everything in the middle of can be treated with some sort of plant that can be discovered becoming actually in a wide range of zones. Societies everywhere throughout the world have been utilizing plants for their therapeutic properties for a considerable length of time, much sooner than drug was packaged and sold in pill structure.

Some of the plants and herbs that can be used to safe life in the wilderness are as follows:

Medicinal use

If there is an occurrence of any disease, a specialist's recommendation is undoubtedly best. However, if there is no doctor available, you may need to depend on Mother Nature's abundance for a stretch before you can look for therapeutic consideration. Following are the medicines which nature provides us:

1. **Aloe Vera:**

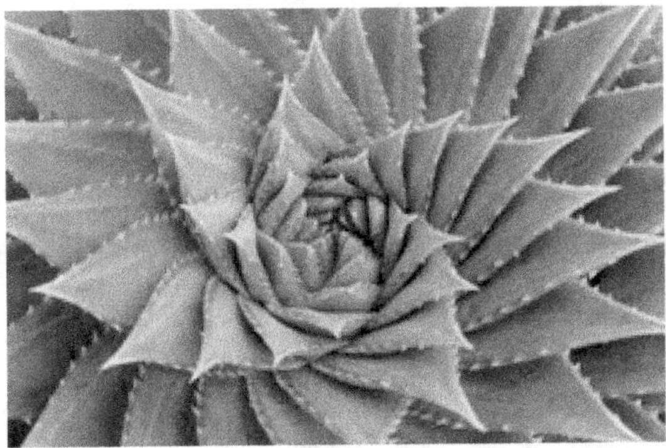

Aloe is a fabulous treatment for skin problems. It is frequently reported that smolders can be mended astoundingly rapidly and the torment diminished rapidly with topical use of Aloe Vera to the blaze zone. And also applying topically, Aloe can likewise be taken inside so it is pretty much as valuable for inner epithelial tissue as it is for the skin. Following are the diseases that Aloe can control:

- Mouth and stomach ulcers

- Lungs and genital tracts.

- Nasal and sinuses

2. Bee Balm:

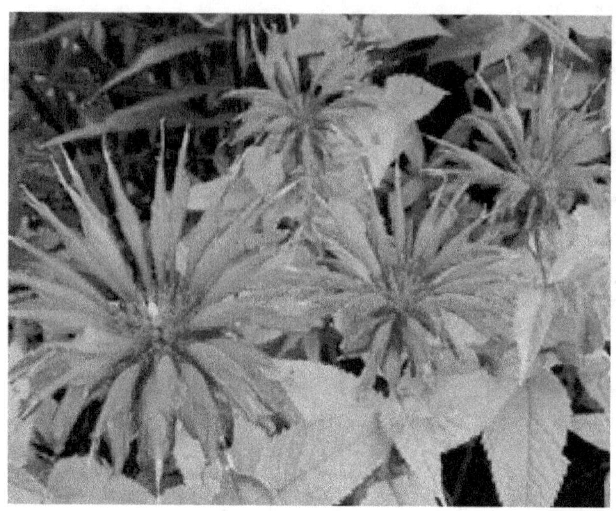

The leaves and flowers of Bee Balm are used for following medicinal purposes:

- Antiseptic

- Carminative

- Diaphoretic

- Diuretic

Furthermore, it is used to cure following disorders:

- Colds

- Headaches

- Sore throat

- Gastric disorders

- Low fevers

- Insomnia

- Flatulence

- Nausea

- Catarrh

- Menstrual pain

Moreover, steam annihilation of Bee Balm is also very helpful while suffering from cold.

3. Blackberries

Blackberry leaf is regularly utilized as a therapeutic herb, yet the root has restorative quality. The young shoots are collected in the spring, peeled and utilized as a part of salads. The most astringent part is the root.

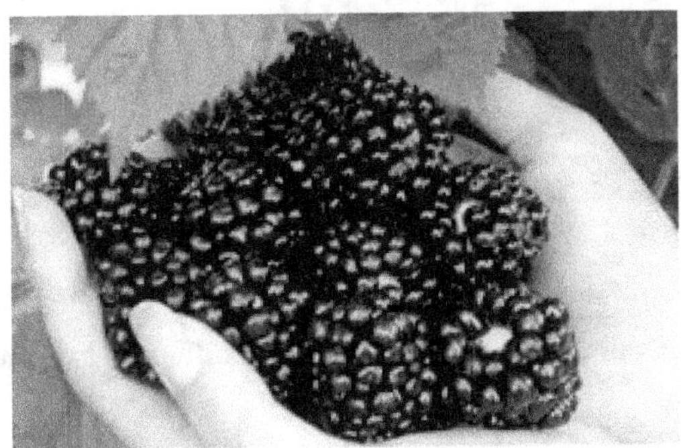

Moreover, they are utilized for the following:

- Sore throats

- Mouth ulcers

- Gum aggravations.

A decoction of the leaves is helpful as a swish in treating thrush furthermore makes a decent broad mouthwash. The nearness of a lot of tannins that give blackberry roots and leaves an astringent impact valuable for treating looseness of the bowels are additionally useful for mitigating sore throats. Moreover, restorative syrup is additionally produced using Blackberry, utilizing the products of the soil bark in nectar for a hack cure.

4. Boneset

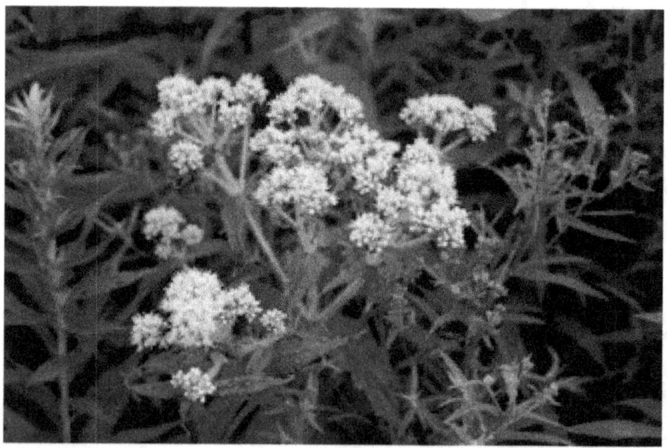

The impact of boneset is slow and persistent. It has great influence on the following:

- Stomach

- Bowels

- Uterus

- Liver

It has been highly regarded as a famous febrifuge, particularly in discontinuous fever, and has been utilized, however less effectively, in typhoid and yellow fevers. It is to a great extent utilized by the Negroes of the Southern United States as a cure in all instances of fever, and in addition for its tonic impacts. As a gentle tonic it is helpful in dyspepsia and general debility, and especially serviceable in the acid reflux of old individuals. The imbuement of 1 OZ of the dried herb to 1 half quart of bubbling water might be taken in wineglassful measurements, hot or icy: for colds and to deliver sweat, it is given hot; as a tonic, frosty.

Food sources:

1. **Acorns:**

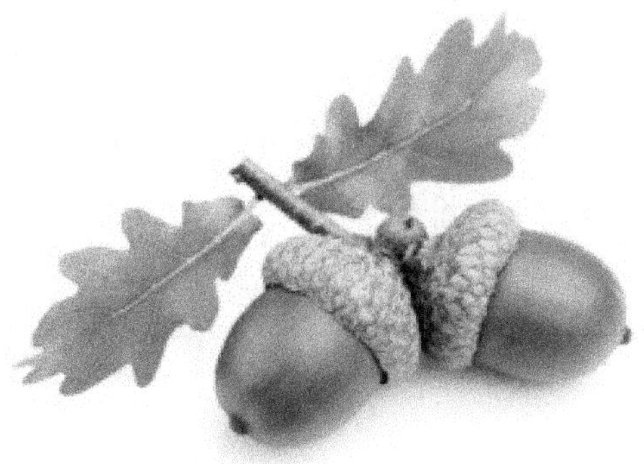

These buds of the oak tree are conventional wellsprings of protein and fat. One can shell and then bubble them, supplanting the water when it becomes brown to dispose of the tannic acid. One might likewise absorb them the running water of a waterway for a day or more

2. Prickly pear cactus:

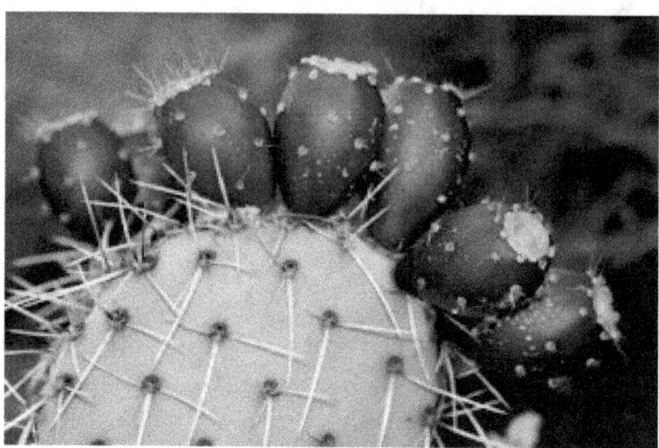

By evacuating the spines and external peel from the youthful stack of the thorny pear, you'll uncover a heavenly and consumable organic product.

3. Purslane:

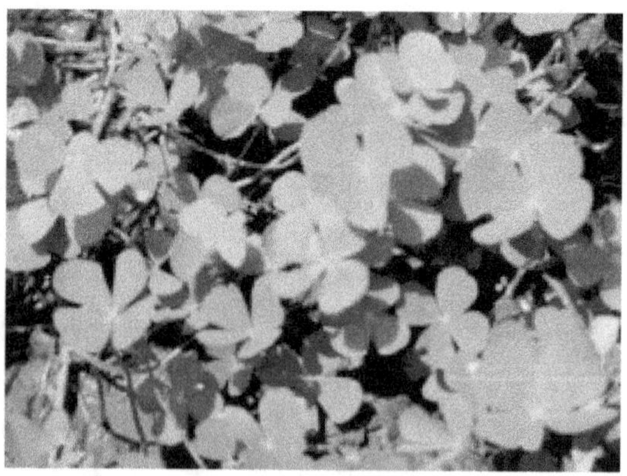

The stems, blossoms, and leaves of this plant contain more omega-3 unsaturated fats than most different greens. Also, here we thought they were just weeds.

Therefore, there are several herbs and plants that can serve the purpose of saving our life in the wilderness. May it as a food resource or as a medicine, plants and herbs can serve the purpose of both.

Chapter 02: Survival Medicine for Fever and Cough

Items produced using botanicals, or plants that are utilized to treat ailments or to keep up the health are called herbal products, botanical items, or phytomedicines. Moreover, the item produced using plants and utilized exclusively for inside use is called a herbal supplement. Furthermore, numerous doctor prescribed medications and over-the-counter prescriptions are additionally produced using plant subsidiaries.

Home grown supplements come in all structures i.e., capsule, dried, powdered, or fluid, and can be utilized as a part of different ways, including:

- Gulped as pills

- Prepared as tea

- Rubbed to the skin as gels

- Added to shower water

The act of utilizing home grown supplements goes back a large number of years. Today, the utilization of home grown supplements is regular among American shoppers. Nonetheless, natural supplements are not for everybody. Since they are not subject to close examination by the FDA, or other representing organizations, the utilization of home grown supplements stays disputable. It is best to counsel your specialist about any indications or conditions you are encountering and to examine the utilization of home grown supplements.

How to cure fever

Many researchers have discovered homemade medicines using herbs and plants that can prove to be useful in curing fever. Some of the approaches that can be used to cure fever are as follow:

1. In order to avoid dehydration use of fluids to a large number is suggested. To flush the sickness away, herbal teas of following herbs are suggested

    - Chamomile

    - Catnip

    - Peppermint

2. Moreover, another way used involves the use of elderberries. Syrup is made out of these berries. This syrup, consequently, helps in curing the disease

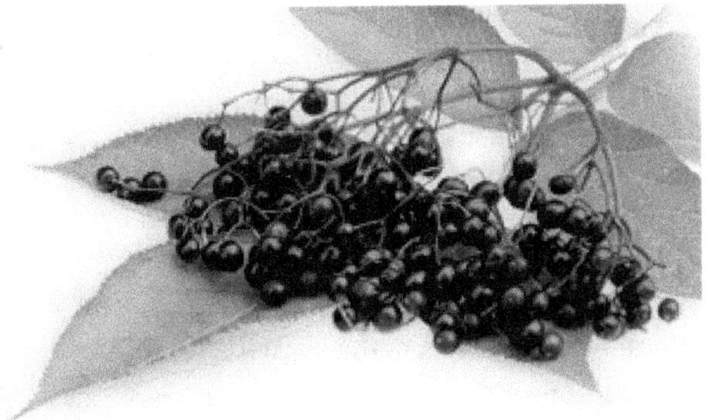

3. Mix some yarrow tea. Interestingly, this herb opens your pores and triggers the sweating that is said to move a fever toward its end. Steep a tablespoon of herb in some crisply bubbled water for 10 minutes. Let it be cooled. Then, drink a glass or two until you begin to sweat.

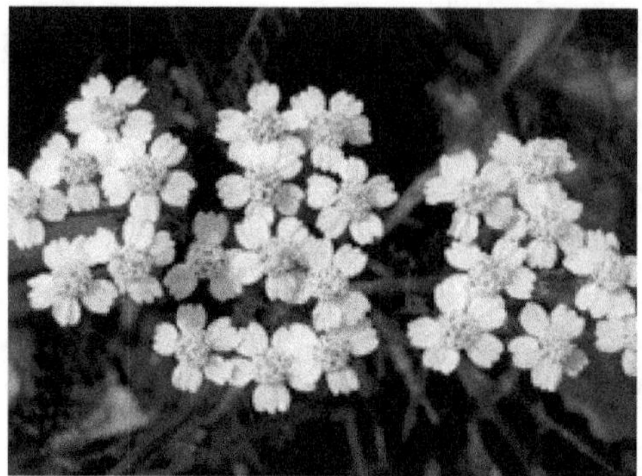

4. Another herb, elderflower, additionally helps you sweat. Additionally, it happens to be useful for different issues connected with influenza and colds, similar to overproduction of bodily fluid. So, to make elderflower tea, blend two teaspoons of the herb in some bubbled water and let it steep for 15 minutes. Strain out the elderflower. Drink three times each day the length of the fever proceeds.

5. Drink some hot ginger tea, which likewise actuates sweating. To make the tea, soak a half-teaspoon minced gingerroot in 1 glass simply boiled water. Strain, then drink.

6. Put some cayenne pepper on your food items whenever you have fever. One of its primary segments is capsaicin, the alarmingly hot fixing that is found in hot peppers. Cayenne makes you sweat furthermore advances fast blood course.

7. White willow has been utilized for a large number of years by Chinese doctors. A tea made of willow bark is maybe the best-known characteristic treatment for fever and torment. A dynamic compound is salicin, which was confined in 1830 and changed over to aspirin, a standout amongst the most well-known cutting edge drugs. The bitter taste of the willow Bark

can be masked with cinnamon, ginger, chamomile, or any of various flavorful herbs

How to cure cold

Before the discovery of anti-biotic, homemade recipes were used in order to cure cold. In order to cure cold following remedial steps must be taken:

1. Get a lot of liquids. It separates your blockage, makes your throat soggy, and avoids dehydration in your body. The vast majority must drink at least ten to eight ounce glasses of liquid consistently.

2. You can relax up your stuffy nose while you take in some steam. Hold your head over a jar of boiling water and inhale gradually through your nose. However, care must be taken while you are inhaling steam. Try not to give the warmth a chance to harm your nose. You can likewise get some alleviation with a humidifier in your room. Moreover, attempt to take some relief from a hot shower.

3. Both saline spray and salt water are used in order to cure cold. In the event that you go the washing course, attempt this formula:

   i. Blend approximately 3 teaspoons of iodide salt and 1 teaspoon of baking soda

   ii. Place the mixture in a sealed shut compartment.

   iii. Now, add 1 teaspoon of the mixture in boiled or refined water.

   iv. Afterwards, fill a syringe with this arrangement and put your head over a bowl. Gently squirt the salt water into your nose. While doing this hold one nostril shut by applying light finger weight while squirting the blend into the other nostril.

v. Let it deplete for some time and after a few moments treat the other nostril.

vi. However, be very careful and make use of refined, sterile, or pre-boiled water when you make this arrangement. Or else you may catch a disease.

vii. Additionally, flush the globule after utilization and leave open to air dry.

Chapter 03: Herbal Antiseptics in the Wilderness

Antiseptic herbs are an operator that slaughters or restrains the development of microorganisms on the outer surfaces of the body and are by and large recognized from natural anti-infection agents that decimate microorganisms inside.

A germicide when connected to wounds and diseases, guarantee that they are perfect and don't deteriorate and have been utilized all through history. A germicide is just a substance that can be put straightforwardly on a slice or contamination to guarantee that it is legitimately spotless and is going to stay perfect as could be expected under the circumstances until the following application.

Germ-killers avoid and balance contamination and the arrangement of discharge by repressing the development of the irresistible life forms. Germs are all around. Some take up habitation in our bodies and benefit us, for example, the amicable microorganisms that colonize the linings of the insides, upper respiratory tract, and lower urinary framework, out-contending terrible organisms, adding to invulnerable safeguard and great processing. Different organisms – infections, microbes, parasites – wreak ruin when they attack our bodies.

Luckily, various herbs have antimicrobial impacts. A considerable lot of these herbs are culinary herbs and flavors, for example, garlic, ginger, thyme, and cinnamon. That implies, regardless of where you will be, you can most likely locate a home grown partner at the neighborhood market. Herbs don't go about as fast or as intensely as medications. For genuine diseases, anti-microbial can spare lives. Then again, herbs produce fewer reactions and don't appear to be connected with the microbial resistance those diseases anti-infection agents.

Various herbs and oils are normal antibacterial and sterile operators and might be utilized as teas, skin washes, made into ointments. Clean herbs will be herbs that contain crucial oils are antibacterial and germ-free. For instance, Thyme is an Antiseptic herb that has been thought about and utilized since old times and the Thymol contained in the herb makes it an astounding germicide and antimicrobial. Numerous individuals are looking to reduce the impacts of artificially based germicides, on their bodies and there are numerous herbs and vital oils that have sterile properties.

Some of the herbal antiseptics that are useful and can help you in the wilderness are as follows:

Cranberry

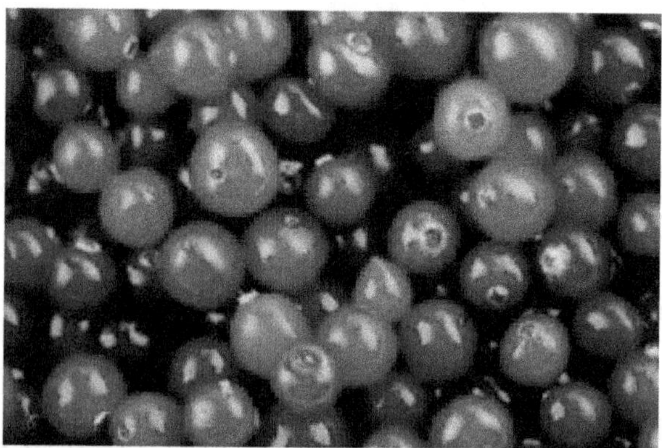

Cranberry also known as Vaccinium macrocarpon is taken as a juice or gathered in tablet structure. It meddles with bacterial adherence to bladder lining, accordingly averting disease. A large portion of the exploration has been in ladies mostly elderly ladies, youthful sexually-dynamic ladies, and pregnant ladies. They are inclined to rehash bladder contaminations. When disease starts, the microbes have effectively connected to the bladder lining. By then, anti-infection agents can clear the contamination quickly and keep microscopic organisms from climbing to the kidneys. For counteractive action, the juice dose utilized as a part of studies reaches from 4 to 32 ounces a day. On the other hand, concentrated juice concentrate can be taken at a dose of one 300-400 milligram tablet, a few times each day. Reactions can incorporate gastrointestinal bombshell. Likewise, concoction constituents of cranberry may hinder the proteins that separate medications, in these way raising blood levels of prescriptions, for instance

- Coumadin

- Valium

- Elavil

- Motrin, and others

Garlic

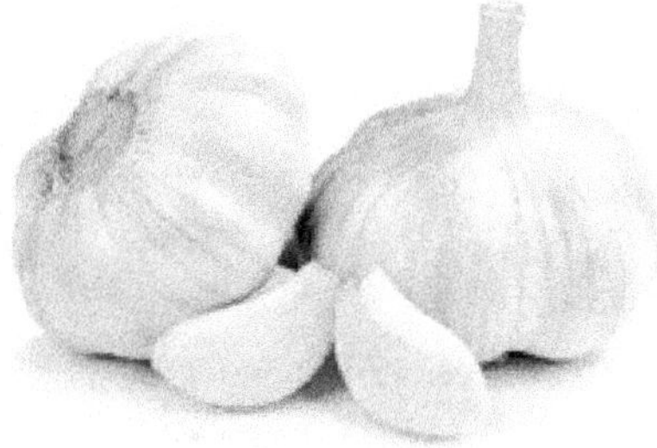

Garlic has antibacterial action against Staphylococcus, Streptococcus, Proteus, Pseudomonas, Mycobacterium, and in addition species connected with loose bowels. However, to some degree strangely, garlic meddles with sickness bringing about microscopic organisms, as opposed to the "amicable" microorganisms, for example, Lactobacillus that colonizes the digestion tracts.

Moreover, garlic is also useful in tackling various species of fungi. Antiviral movement incorporates influenza An and B, rhinovirus, cytomegalovirus, HIV, rotavirus, herpes simplex infection 1 and 2, and a few species that results in pneumonia. According to a particular research those people who use a garlic supplement commencing November through February had few chances of getting sick due to fewer than all those people who use pills. Other Allium types (chives, leeks, onions) have antimicrobial drive as well.

A significant part of the data related to garlic's antimicrobial strength instigates from lab ponders. A smaller amount is thought about in what manner garlic arrangements graft in people contaminated by means of these "bugs." The similar can be assumed in regards to the greater part of alternate herbs recorded beneath. Heat neutralizes garlic's antimicrobial elements. Therefore, it's preeminent to devour it crude or as a pill that promises a specific amount of allicin. On the off chance that you spread over garlic topically as an adhesive, ensure the skin using olive or any other type of oil, spread with dressing or clean material, and evacuate following 60 minutes.

Marshmallow root:

Marshmallow is most normally used to straightforwardness sore throats and dry hacks. The Marshmallow plant contains polysaccharides that have antitussive, adhesive, and antibacterial properties. In light of this, marshmallow soothingly affects aggravated films in the mouth and throat when ingested orally, particularly a sore throat. The antitussive properties diminish dry hacking and avoid further aggravation.

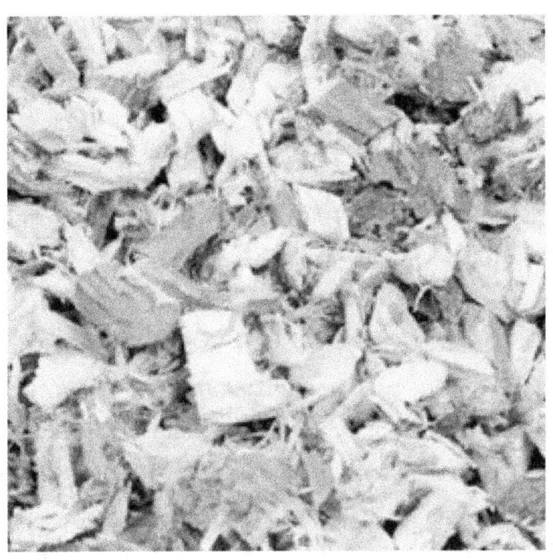

According to the research, marshmallow has been utilized to treat certain digestive issue, including acid reflux, heartburn, ulcerative colitis, stomach ulcers and Crohn's sickness. The system by which it calms sore throats applies to gastrointestinal mucosa too and consistent utilization of marshmallow can help with the agony of ulcerative colitis and Crohn's, and keep stomach ulcers from puncturing. Marshmallow concentrate is now and again added to creams and used to treat provocative skin conditions, for example, dermatitis and contact dermatitis. Extra uses are right now being explored. Marshmallow might be a useful guide to radiologic esophageal examination. There is conditional proof that marshmallow may likewise help with respiratory issue, for example, asthma. Scientists may soon test marshmallow as a characteristic contrasting option to glucose administration in diabetes.

Chapter 04: Common Ailments and Their Herbal Cures

As our way of life is getting techno-astute, we are moving far from nature. While we can't escape from nature since we are a piece of nature. What nature has put away in for us we have not yet completely discovered? This can irritate point with people. Certain European and Oriental nations have been investigating the utilization of herbs and has been by and by since the hundreds of years. Awesome work has been done which escaped the regular man's scope and information .With life on tech-course for each person in the 21st century human sufferings are turning out with various names .The essential herbs have the answer, the general key is no symptoms and powerful cures. The cures are in a state of harmony with nature which is the greatest in addition to point where no other drug can guarantee these actualities. The brilliant certainty is utilization of home grown medicines is autonomous of any age bunches.

Following are some of the common ailments along with their herbal cure are as follows:

Skin problems

1. **Burns:**

    i. **Honey:** This is particularly useful for serious smolders. It will stop disease, invigorate skin recovery and keep the blazed region sodden. Nectar is preferred for smolders over about every single medicinal intercession, notwithstanding for severe singeing.

    ii. **Prickly pear cactus pads:** Wear gloves to hold the cushions while utilizing a sharp blade to delicately filet the outside skin off the cushions. You will be left with disgusting, oval stack of plant matter. Place the cushions specifically on the smolder and wrap the injury. For sunburn, rub the cushions on the influenced region.

2. Cuts and scratches.

Each one of us experiences sharp edges may it is a paper cut or a knife cut, regularly again and again. Here's the way to handle the consequences.

i. **Wound powder:** My natively constructed wound powder stops the dying, dries out the injury, represses disease and empowers recuperating. I by and large utilize a gauze the primary day and afterward leave the injury open a while later

ii. **Honey:** Stop utilizing the injury powder following a couple days and switch to nectar. It's viable against all known medication safe microscopic organisms and truly speeds recuperating. Simply cover the injury with nectar, swathe, and change the dressing every day.

iii. **Wound balm:** Use a mix of berberine plants, Siberian elm bark, rosemary leaves, dark walnut bodies, comfrey root, oregano leaves, and dried thyme. Include a quarter-container each of the generally ground herbs to a preparing dish and blend. Spread the mix with around a quarter-inch olive oil, cover the dish, and prepare overnight in a stove on its most reduced warmth setting. In the morning, let the blend cool. Press out and afterward warm the oil. Blend in finely cleaved or ground beeswax — 2 ounces for each measure of mixed oil — and let melt. To check hardness, put a drop of treatment on a plate and hold up until the ointment cools. It ought to stay strong however dissolve following a second of preceding it with your finger.

3. Rashes:

Rashes come in numerous structures, so medications will shift. Here are a couple of them.

i. **For hives:** Put on a tincture of Echinacea angustifolia root topically, utilizing a cotton ball to regulate it to the influenced territories. Take a half-teaspoon of the tincture inside every hour or so also.

ii. **For toxic substance ivy:** Jewelweed balm is ideal. Great added substances are calendula blooms, chamomile blossoms and Siberian elm bark, all of which will calm skin. Include some other herbs you need, however utilize the ethereal parts of a jewelweed plant for half of the dried herbs by weight. At that point, take after the same procedure as above for making the injury treatment.

4. **Stings and chomps**:

Utilize thorny pear as you would for blazes or Echinacea as you would for hives.

Intestinal Upsets

1. **Loose bowels:**

Any firmly astringent plant will work for customary looseness of the bowels. Blackberry root, the primary standby utilized for millennia, is greatly compelling. Krameria root, more seasoned pine needles just pulled off the tree, and wild (Geranium maculatum) are all extremely supportive for direction. To utilize, generally slash or crush your preferred dried herb. Add 1 ounce to a quart jug that can take warmth, and load with boiling point water. Spread the invention and let it soak overnight (or for two hours in the event that you truly can hardly wait). Drink it all through the following day. Rehash as required.

2. **Gastric disorder:**

To begin, make juice of 1 beet, 1 bit of green cabbage (about the extent of a medium carrot), 3 carrots, 4 stalks of celery and 4 leaves of crisp plantain (Plantago spp.). Plantain is a typical plant you can generally discover developing in front yards, and is random to the banana of the same name. Cabbage and plantain are the most essential fixings; however they don't taste great without anyone else. Alternate fixings will enhance the taste while helping your adrenal organs, liver and insusceptible framework. Drink this squeeze each morning for breakfast, have cereal for lunch, and have whatever you need for supper. Touchy gut disorder will clear decently quickly on this regimen.

Chapter 05: Precautions to Use Peppers Survival Medicine

To begin with, herbal medicines are used by multiple people which the following purposes:

- Anti-microbial

- Anti-bacterial

- Iodine wash

- Anti-viral

Every measurement of anti-biotic should be weighed deliberately, since re-supply won't come, in the lack of supplies decent homemade information may spare the life of somebody you adore.

Nonetheless, it is important that given the sheer number of home grown meds, and impressive heterogeneity inside and between brands, it is not possible to assess all items for their pharmacology. Albeit some natural pharmaceuticals have had broad examination, a large portion of them have not. Indeed, even those that have been moderately very much concentrated frequently have little data in extraordinary populaces, for example, pediatric, pregnant or lactating ladies, or geriatric populaces, and subsequently, alert ought to be utilized while prescribing natural medications to these populaces.

Some of the side effects of using peppers survival medicine are as follows:

1. Skin allergies:

Topical home grown antifungal and antibacterial operators, for example, tea tree oil and lavender are capable of causing rashes or skin disturbance, particularly if utilized at full quality. Before utilizing any topical home grown item, attempt a skin patch test. Place a little measure of the item within the elbow on one arm as it were. Hold up a couple days. On the off chance that the range stays clear, continue with utilizing the home grown item

2. Dizziness:

Everybody's body is distinctive, and some individuals are more delicate to herbs than other individuals. Herbs used to treat uneasiness, melancholy and a sleeping disorder may bring about extreme daytime lethargy in specific people. These herbs incorporate chamomile, valerian and kava, with valerian and kava being the in all probability offenders. Abstain from driving or utilizing apparatus until you're certain of the impacts of the herb.

3. Photosensitivity:

People taking herbal medicines treat despondency or uneasiness may discover their skin turning out to be more delicate to the sun. They may blaze all the more effortlessly. Commonly, reasonable haired and light-cleaned Caucasians have the most astounding occurrence of photosensitivity, yet this home grown reaction is thankfully uncommon. Common instances of photosensitivity happen when individuals take high dosages of herbal medicine, or take it over a drawn out stretch of time. In the case of taking herbal medicine, maintain a strategic distance from an excess of sun presentation

However, if someone desires to eliminate the danger of getting harmed by using dangerous herbs or plants as medicines, then he must adopt following precautionary measures:

Learn to differentiate between harmful and harmless plants:

Firstly, one must learn how to differentiate between those plants which are harmful and which one of them are harmless. This very approach will help the person choosing the plants for medicinal purposes. If a person is unaware about the plants, then he might get confused and use a wrong herb. This can cause various allergies and can even lead to death

1. Never utilize any plant without the validness of its character:

Secondly, any plant must not be utilized before its complete recognizable proof. This may represent a risk to one's wellbeing. Hence, a plant must not be utilized before its 100% distinguishing proof

2. Do not get confused between plants:

Thirdly, multiple plants look similar to one another. However, not all of them are useable. Therefore, never get confused by the deceiving looks of the plant

3. Avoid excessive use of the herbs:

Fourthly, one should avoid the excessive use of plants and herbs. If one uses the herb in an excessive quantity, then it might cause damage to the person using the herb. In the event that you utilize home grown supplements, take after mark guidelines deliberately and utilize the endorsed dose as it were. Never surpass the suggested dose, and search out data about who ought not to take the supplement.

4. Look for reactions:

If any symptoms, for example, sickness, unsteadiness, cerebral pain, or furious stomach, happen, diminish the measurements or quit taking the home grown supplement

5. Be ready for an unfavorably responses:

A serious hypersensitive response can bring about trouble relaxing. If any unlikely event occurs, rush to the emergency to avoid any harm.

6. Do some research:

Research about the organization whose herbs you are taking. All home grown supplements are not made equivalent, and it is best to pick a respectable maker.

Moreover, following things must be checked before using any homemade medicine:

- Has the manufacturer put some effort in developing the herbal product or if he is employing the some one's research.

- Does the item make abnormal or difficult to demonstrate claims?

- Does the item mark give data about the institutionalized equation, reactions, fixings, bearings, and safeguards?

- Is the provided data clear and simple to peruse?

Conclusion

To put in a nutshell, plants and herbs are an efficient source of medicines. This book will expound upon all of those perspectives that will help an individual and guide him about the herbal medicines. Moreover, living out in the wild, you'll keep running over an extensive variety of remedial plants and helpful herbs that can be used for different purposes, the length of you know where to look and how to use them. Various plants are profitable for sustenance, and can be used as pharmaceutical too. Plants can be used to alleviate an extensive variety of ailments. Everything from skin rash, joint irritation, cool, fever, detachment of the insides, cerebral pains, and everything amidst can be treated with some kind of plant that can be found turning out to be really in an extensive variety of zones. Social orders all over the place all through the world have been using plants for their helpful properties for an impressive time span, much sooner than medication was bundled and sold in pill structure. Regardless, it is essential that given the sheer number of home developed meds, and great heterogeneity inside and between brands, it is unrealistic to evaluate all things for their pharmacology. But some normal pharmaceuticals have had wide examination, an extensive part of them have not. Surely, even those that have been decently especially focused as often as possible have little information in remarkable peoples. Therefore, the book includes in itself all the precautions that are necessary

25 Best Herbs and Herbal Mixes to Use As Herbal Remedies for Health and Healing

Introduction: Flower Power!

The use of herbs for healing is a global tradition that all of humanity shares. For those of us who can understand the powerful healing that can be obtained from the roots of the ground, herbal remedies our more than a treatment or recreational hobby, they are determined way of life. Those that engage in naturopathy (healing from nature) develop a distinctive philosophy and can-do attitude when it comes to illness and disease.

For those that have learned to treat their ailments with the herbal remedies that nature provides us for free. And the historic precedent for this natural treatment is long; the very father of medicine Hippocrates was a staunch supporter of herbal therapy, setting up his own herbal clinics in his own heyday of 400 BC! He sang the praises of these herbs his entire practice.

In fact, one of the most famous quotes attributed to this ancient physician is, "Nature Cures, not the Physician." It seems the father of medicine knew full well the source of his healing prowess. This was a theme that carried on through Aristotle and other Greek physicians that knew full well the tremendous resource that roots, fruits, and flowers can provide.

Chapter 1: Aches and Pains. Herbal Remedies for what Ails You!

We all suffer from aches and pains from time to time, the technical term for it is "Myalgia" which roughly translates as "Pain in the Muscles". One of the most common of these aches and pains you may have heard of is "Fibromyalgia". This is a particularly devastating disorder of the musculoskeletal system, characterized by wide spread pain throughout the body followed by deep seated fatigue.

Fibromyalgia could be said to be the mother load of all aches and pains and it is caused by an imbalance of chemicals and a disruption in which the brain processes pain signals. The good news is, medicinal herbs can help to treat and possibly reverse even this devastating illness. Because medicinal herbs can work to refine and readjust those ailing pain processors of the brain, allowing you to rework how your body interprets external stressors.

At its core a disorder such as Fibromyalgia is just a magnification of what all of us face as our body gets older and discomfort increases. It is this pain felt deep inside our muscle tissue that leads to a lot of discomfort as our body gets older and more worn down later in life.

But whether it's that chronic bad back, that nagging headache or your arthritic wrists, the human body, like a machine, gets wore out from prolonged use. Unlike your car however, many of your aches and pains can be fixed without a $1000 overhaul of your engine! So without footing a major bill, let's go down the list of some of the best herbs for what ails you!

Ginger

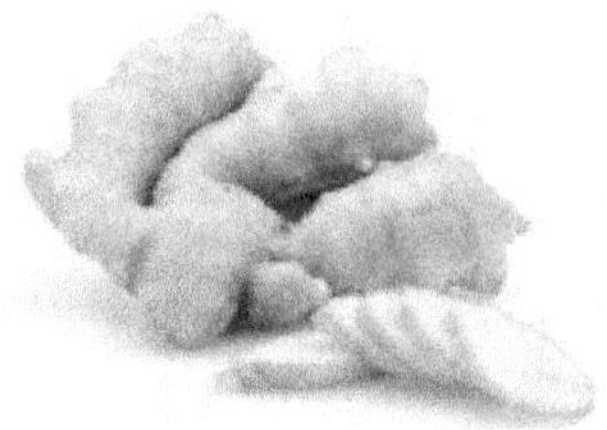

Ginger extract has been proven to have a positive effect on most joint and muscle pain. The main active agent within ginger that aids in this are called "phytochemcials" an ingredient that works to lessen inflammation. Just grind ginger into powder and rub it into your aching joints for instant relief. You can also put into tasty teas and drink it for a powerful healing effect on your aches and pains.

Tumeric

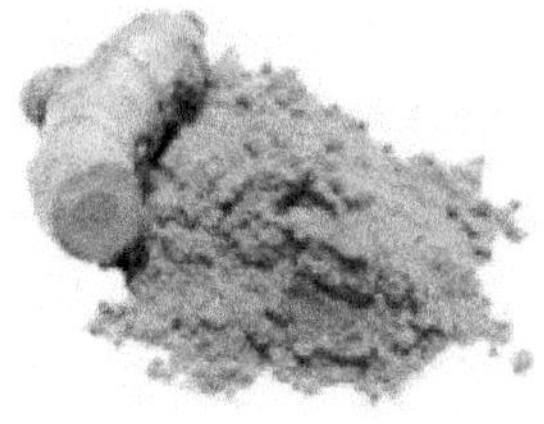

For those of you who suffer from chronic arthritis, Tumeric could be your best friend. Similar to Ginger, Tumeric works as a natural inflammation reducer. It's main ingredient "curcurmin" has powerful anti-inflammatory properties that ease their way right into arthritic wrists and joints. Tumeric is an ancient herb with a long history of practice.

Whatever aches and pains anyone has, Tumeric holds the promise to eliminate it. Along with arthritis Tumeric is also known to reduce heartburn, so whether you are suffering from a back ache or a stomach ache, it is still well worth a try. Tumeric is also a quite tasty seasoning for a wide variety of foods so don't be afraid to experiment with this pain neutralizing herb.

Devil's Claw

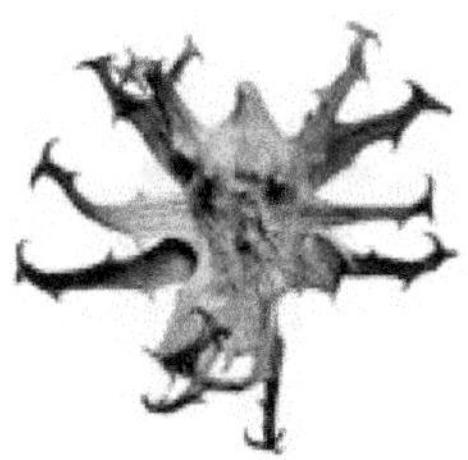

While this herb may not have a very appealing name, when it comes to the healing properties of this herb's, there is nothing devilish about it! Herbalists have used Devil's Claw to treat aches and pains for many generations. And for those that suffer from back aches in particular, this herb holds much promise. Because when Devil's Claw is ground into powder and applied in a compress to the lower back, it can provide great relief to back pain sufferers.

Hailing from South Africa this herb has been sought out from far and wide in order to avoid a visit to the chiropractor! And don't just take our word for it; there is documented research to back this up! In a controlled study in 2002 227 patients were administered this herb to treat back and hip pain, and out of these 227 patients, 70% of the participants reported improvement and even more than that an increase in mobility.

The active ingredients in this medicinal herb have the ability to loosen up even the most stubborn of joints and muscles to relieve your aches and pains. Devil's Claw can be found at most health food and herbal stores, and it can be grown for individual practice as well. So if you can get past this medicinal herb's strange name and appearance you will have a great asset on your hands when it comes to the battle against aches and pains.

Valerian Root

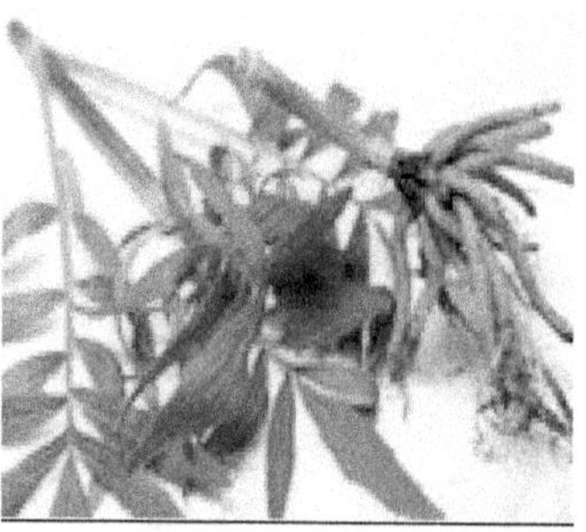

Valerian Root is a wonder herb and it has a long list of benefits, and one of the lesser known of these positives is the way in which this herb can relieve leg cramps and muscle spasms. Just apply this herb to the skin and let the soothing begin! Studies have shown that this root can work directly on the nervous system as a pain reliever. Valeria Root is popular for a wide range of musculoskeletal problems.

This root is also widespread, grown and found in large amounts in Europe, Mexico and India alike. Typical use of this herb involves either grinding it into powder, extracting essential oil from the root, or boiling the plant for use in beverages. I usually boil the root in a hot tea when I administer the herb to myself after a hectic day, allowing my aching muscles to relax!

Burdock Root

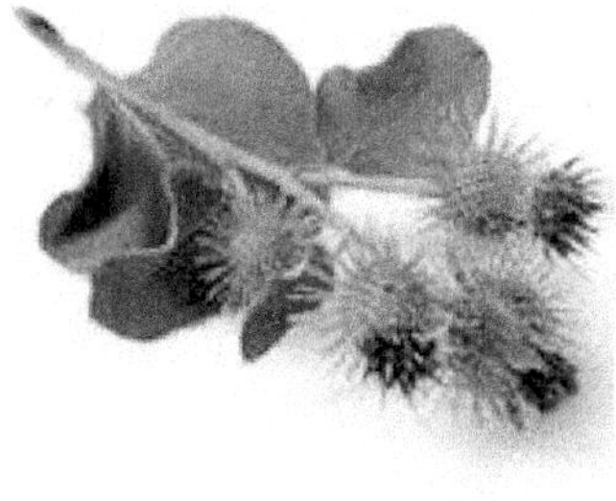

A dry and oily root that is known for lubricating and moistening even the stiffest of joints, Burdock is best used when ground into a fine paste or powder and applied directly to your aches and pains for maximum effect. The plant is easily recognizable by its wavy-edged, and arrow shaped leaves.

The flowers of the plant are usually purple or pink and appear in burr like clusters and can grow an astounding 2 meters tall. Burdock can be found scattered across northern climates all across the globe and is most prevalent in the late spring and early summer months.

The root of the Burdock plant can be ground into a powder and applied to the joints or a liquid can be extracted by boiling it. The essential oil extracted from this herb is very potent however so when attempting to use it just remember that old adage; a little dab will do you! You can use all of these great medicinal herbs to kick those pesky aches and pains straight to the curb!

Chapter 2: Boost Your Immune System with Herbal Remedies

Our immune system is our most important tool of survival, without it we couldn't even step outside and face day. Just like in the famous movie, "The Bubble Boy" without our built in protection from contaminates, we would literally have to live in a bubble just to keep from being compromised.

Your immune system uses an army of white blood cells to stave off invasion by the harmful bacteria and viruses that we encounter on a daily basis. Any given day of the week your body produces about 1000 million white blood cells. Out of this main army of cells, highly specialized white blood cells of your immune system known as "Macrohages" literally go on patrol seeking and destroying any germs that enter your system.

It is through our Immune System's constant filtering and elimination of harmful elements that we can remain healthy. Having that said, wouldn't it be great if we could give our immune system a little jumpstart every now and then. Well my friends, then look no further than nature, because there are quite a few herbs that can play a pivotal role in our immune health.

Echinacea

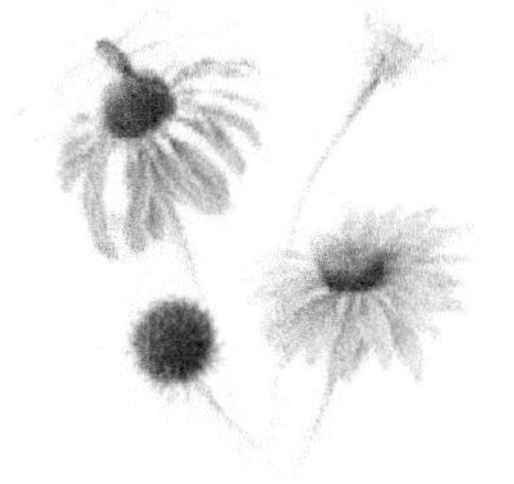

A member of the daisy family, this herb has astounding anti-biotic and even anti-viral properties and we would really be amiss not to mention it. Many herbal enthusiasts make a powerful tea and tonic from its extracted oil and use it to boost their immune system against bacteria, germs, and viruses. Just the aroma of this herb alone is enough to open the nasal passages. Moderate doses of this herb can treat even the worst cold and allergy symptoms as well as being beneficial to upper respiratory tract infections.

Reishi

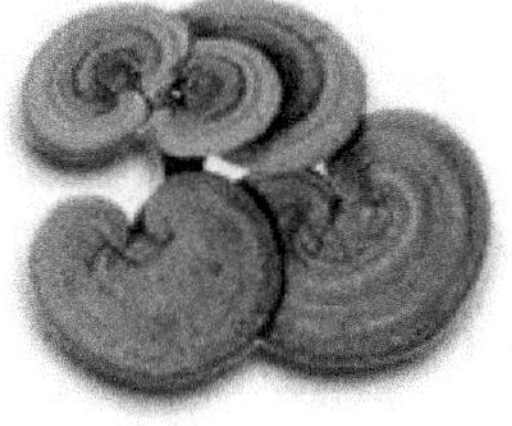

Also known as Ganoderma, Reishi is a bitter mushroom that has been used in Chinese herbal medicine for thousands of years. This herb has been shown to not only improve the immune system, but to improve longevity in general. Its heavy antioxidant properties have been used to treat everything from cancer to urinary tract infections.

Known as an "immune modulator" the properties of this magical mushroom work to fine tune and regulate your immune system. There is no special preparation required for this herbal remedy, really all you have to do is eat it and experience the results. In no time you will see that regular consumption of this herbal mushroom will improve blood flow and enhance your overall immune health.

Astragalus

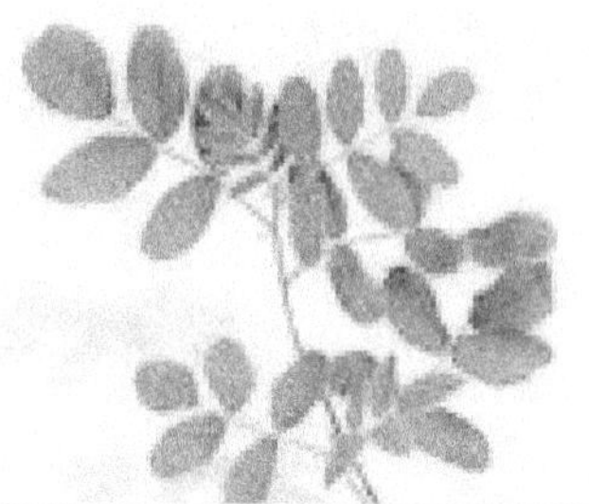

Another Chinese herb, Astragalus has been used in the Orient for thousands of years as herbal medicine. Sold by the boatload as dried root slices, this herb is still used to this very day as a powerful immune booster. Traditionally this herb has been served up in warm soups such as chicken broth.

An idea that seems to lend some credence to your mother's assertion that all a bad cold needs is a good bowl of chicken noodle soup! In fact as an immune system trigger, Astragalus has been found to be so powerful that it can directly activate the marrow of our lymph tissue and stimulate the development of our active immune cells.

These roots can be ground into powder and oil can be extracted to use in aroma therapy or as soothing creams for an herbal massage. The leaves of this plant can also be used to make teas that are good for the throat and empowering to the rest of our bodily function. This is an amazing herb and its benefits are well worth the trouble of obtaining it.

Cat's Claw

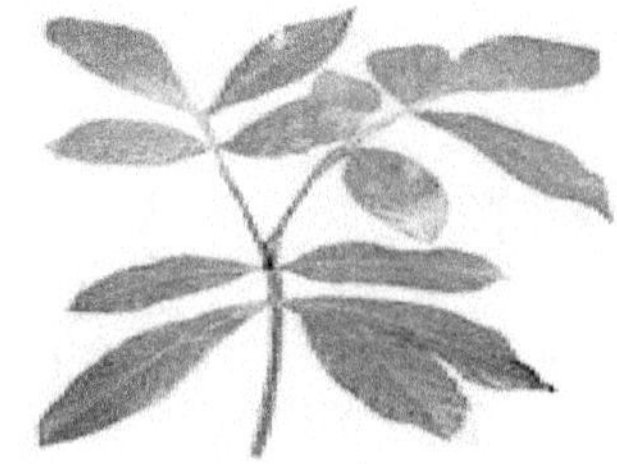

This woodsy vine is native to the rain forests of the Amazon in South America. Similar to the "Devil's Claw", the strange name of this herb comes from its somewhat odd appearance of curved, claw shaped thorns that look almost like a cat's claw. (If the shoe fits wear it right?)

But regardless of what it looks like the roots of this medicinal herb have been used for over 2000 years by the indigenous tribes of South America for their healing and immune boosting properties. When used properly this herb is known to significantly increase the white blood cell count and regulate the immune system.

These herbs have been recommended as an alternative therapy for both Aids and Cancer. For Cancer patients in particular, this herb has shown promise in helping to ease some of the harshness of chemotherapy. The root is typically served up in tea or ground into a powder that can be rubbed on the skin. All of the herbs mentioned in this chapter are all significant ways in which you can boost your immune system.

Chapter 3: Herbal Remedies for Anxiety and Depression

We live in a fast paced world, but unfortunately as we try our best to get ahead in our careers and social lives much of our peace of mind is left behind! In the hustle and bustle of the modern world we tend to neglect crucial aspects of wellness and stress free living.

And as a result much of the developed world, despite its technological progress, is in the full blown grip of anxiety and depression. And as stress levels rise millions of people around the globe are looking for new ways to relieve their sadness, worry, fears and frustration. But before you turn to more pharmaceutical meds, let's take a look at what nature can provide us to remedy our anxiety and depression.

Passionflower

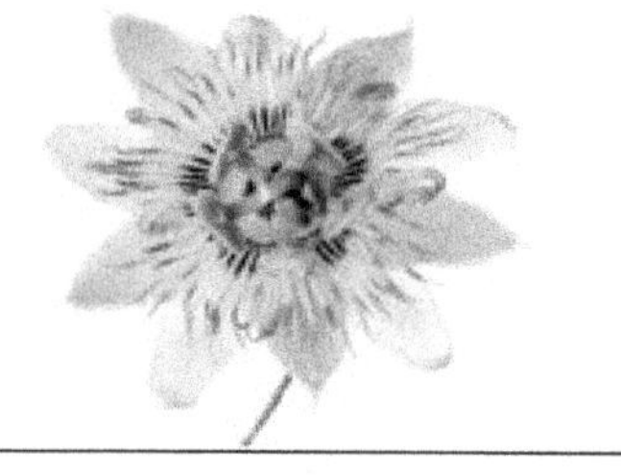

Once again demonstrating the power of the flower, this medicinal herb has been shown to work just as well as many pharmaceutical prescribed anxiety meds. With its remarkable healing of depression, irritability, anxiety and agitation, this is certainly a flower to be passionate about.

You may have also have heard of passionflower as quite a popular beverage at your local star bucks. Yes just ask your barista, because they know full well that this flower most definitely has the power to make you feel pretty darn good!

Lavender

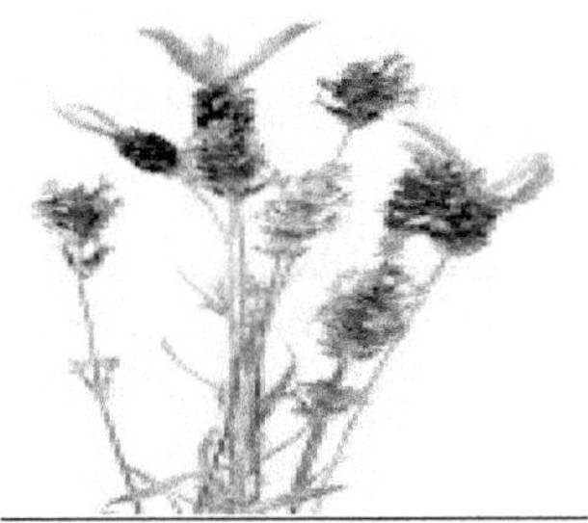

Lavender has been proven time and time again to be quite an effective agent against anxiety. An added bonus to this is that unlike other herbal treatments for anxiety such as Chamomile, Lavender does not have the side effect of making you sleepy.

There is no drowsiness reported from the ingestion of Lavender, so this herbal medicine can be taken at all hours of the day, allowing you to still stay alert and fresh. Lavender is often extracted as an essential oil and massaged into the skin or even worn as perfume, allowing its aromatic healing and stress relief to take full effect.

Kava

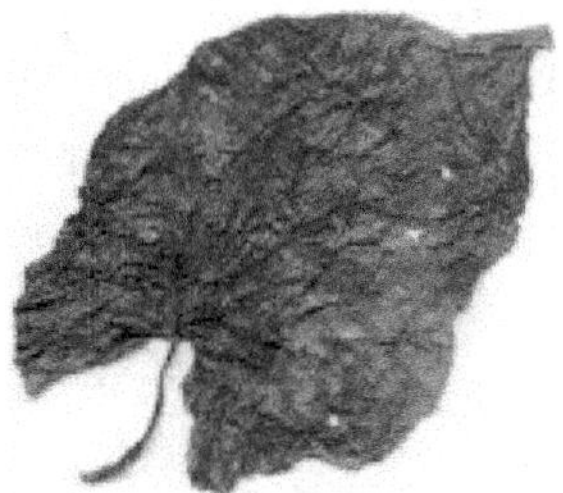

Kava, or as it is known in the islands; Kava! Kava! The Polynesians of the Pacific have used the roots of the Kava plant for thousands of years as a means to treat social anxiety. Viewed as a safer and less destructive version of alcohol, the boiled roots of this plant can be drank as an instantly relaxing tea.

Kava relaxes the body as a mild sedative but without interruption of cognitive function, so unlike alcohol you can relax with this herb without losing any control or quality of your everyday routine. Unlike alcohol Kava has not shown any addictive properties so use can easily be discontinued.

As great as some of the benefits of this medicinal herb are however, Kava is not without its controversy. And despite its proven benefit it's long term use has also been associated with liver damage, causing it to be banned in Europe. Kava is however still available in the United States at most health food and wellness shops.

Ashwagandha

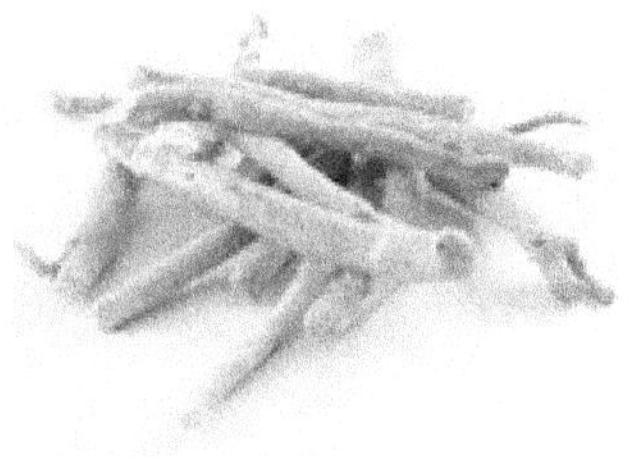

This medicinal herb has been a powerful part of Ayurdvedic medicine for centuries. Known as an "adaptogen" because of its ability to help the human body adapt, this herb gives you what you need to be able to get through stressful situations. The roots of this plant have a powerful effect on stress, gently soothing the body and the mind. The best way to take this herb is to boil the roots of it in teas and directly drink the benefit.

Lemon Balm

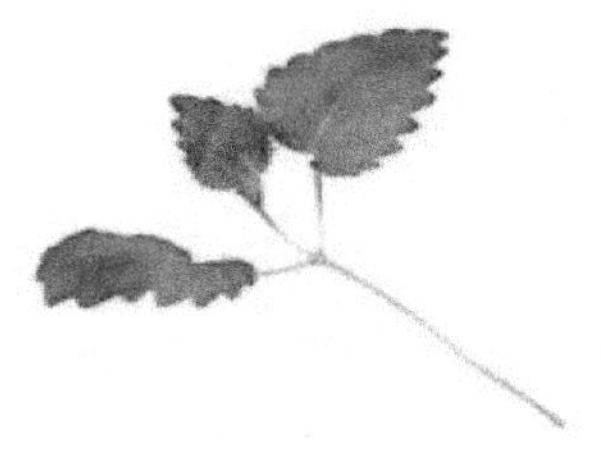

A medicinal herb from the Mint family, this herb has been shown to engender calmness for up to 6 hours after its use. This herb was used in the Middle Ages as a kind of tonic to reduce stress. It was a rather ubiquitous part of medieval society found in medicine, food, and even alcohol.

Today, this herb is still rather prevalent, and is used in many parts of the globe. It can often be found combined with Chamomile (another known calming agent) and boiled in teas and other soothing hot drinks. It is from the leaves that most of the medicinal aspect of this plant is derived.

The leaves can be applied directly to the skin as a cream or it can be reduced to a powder and absorbed through soothing baths. This herb is native Europe but can now be found growing just about anywhere in the world. The plant itself grows to about 2 feet high and is easily recognizable for its bright yellow flowers.

St. John's Wort

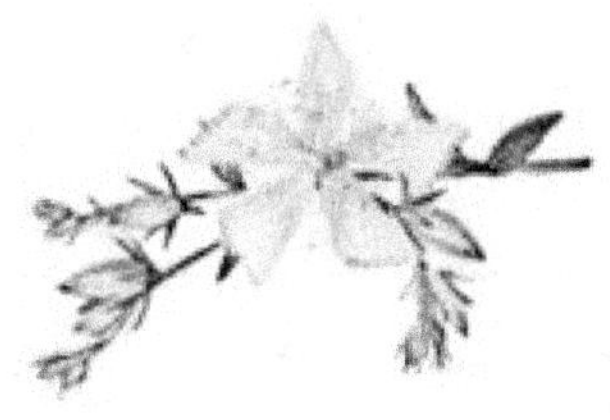

A friend had recommended this one to me years ago after my dad had passed away. She told me that it would help elevate my mood on the days that my grief had become too overwhelming. And while this obviously isn't a cure for grief in itself, it did help me out of the deepest aspects of depression.

St. Johns Wort is grown naturally in much of Europe, Asia, and North Africa. It has been used by Europeans especially to treat mod disturbances such as depression for quite some time. This herb has been associated with boosting Serotonin levels.

Serotonin is the body's "happy chemical" that directly bonds with the neurotransmitters of our brain to help make us feel good. Many people who have chronic depression suffer from a chemical imbalance in which they are lacking in this chemical. A medicinal herb like St. John's Wort helps to correct this imbalance and make you feel better.

Safron

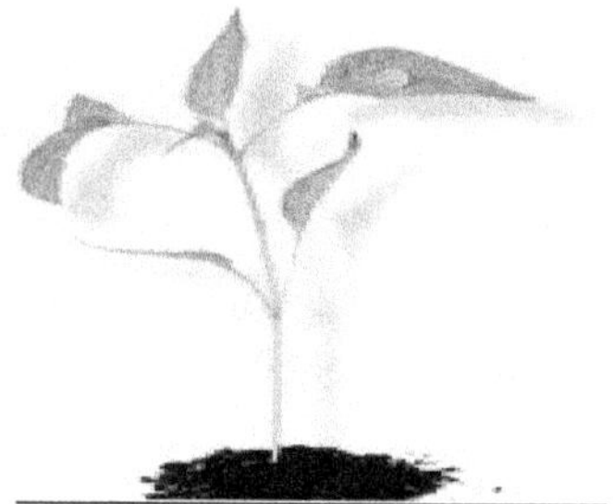

This herb may not look too flashy, but it is a well known depression fighter. This plant is derived from the iris family and is found all over the globe. It is the end of the stem that is most often used to treat mild to moderate forms of depression. Safron is typically prepared by taking the strands of the plant and then either boiling them or grinding them into powder. Just sprinkle a little over your food or use it to make a relaxing tea. One great herbal remedy among many that will get you to feel right once again!

Chapter 4: Herbal Weight Loss

Our expanding waist lines have become an epidemic and every single day new methods of weight loss appear before us. But moving beyond diet fads and get thin quick gimmicks, let's take a look at what some good medicinal herbs can do to aid us in our weight loss challenge and diet routine. Because whether you are trying to lose weight or just live life a little bit healthier, there is bound to be an herb that can help you get there.

Grapefruit

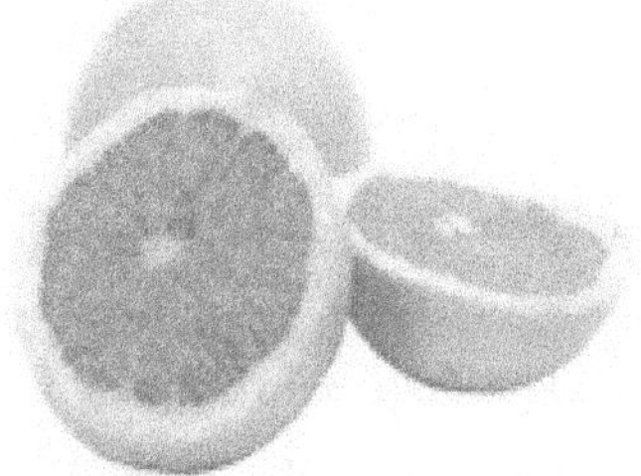

At first glance you may not think of the common grapefruit as a medicinal herb, but looks can be deceiving. Because it so happens that the Grapefruit contains a powerful fat burning molecule that helps the body's liver to burn up fat rather than storing it. This transference from storing fat to actually burning it is the key to any successful weight loss regimen.

Moderate Grapefruit consumption is also known to balance out the blood sugar levels of the body and helps to aid in the body's metabolism. It is the juice of the Grape fruit in particular that acts as such a great weight loss agent. So a good way to jumpstart your weight loss routine would be to take this herb and blend it into a juice, and drink up to your weight loss!

Kelp Seaweed

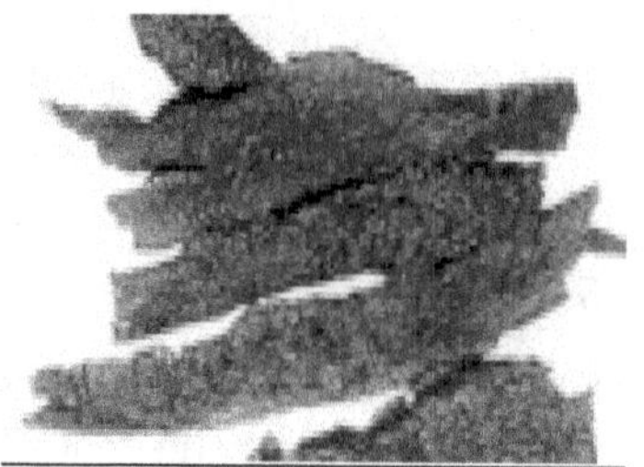

Known by the Japanese for many years, this herb has been scooped out of the ocean and added to the diet to help aid weight loss. The reason why Kelp can work to help us lose weight is due to the fact that it is rich in iodine. This powerful chemical directly interacts with your thyroid gland helping to jumpstart your metabolism.

Dried and powdered Kelp can be used as an extra seasoning additive to sprinkle on your food. The taste is fairly rich and it can be put on just about anything. Kelp soups and salads are a particular favorite and easy to prepare. Kelp can be found at most grocery stores and health food centers, so don't be afraid to serve yourself up a helping of kelp, and just watch that old weight come falling off!

Prickly Pear

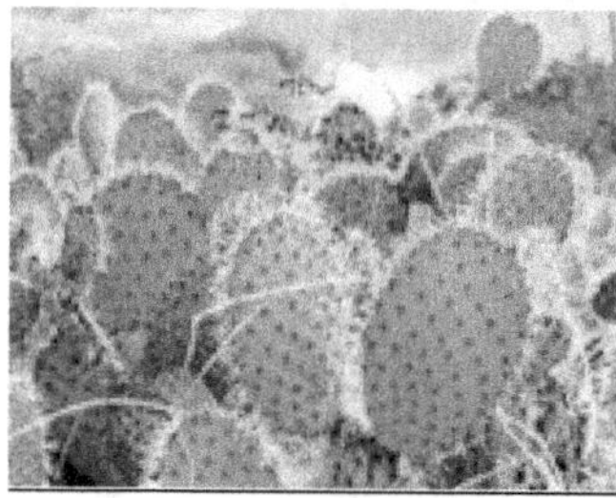

Prickly Pear hails from the cactus family and can be found growing wild all throughout Mexico. Long known to the Native Americans tribes of Mexico and Central America, this Prickly Pear has now gained some traction in much wider circles and has been used to treat diabetes, lower cholesterol and manage weight loss.

This fruit naturally has high antioxidant levels that tend to aid in weight loss. One of the great assets of this Pear is its use as a cleanser because ingestion of this herb helps to reduce the body's water retention and cleanses the system of excess liquid. This initial water loss alone is a great and helpful aid in beginning your overall weight loss regimen.

This fruit can be found at most health food stores and can be grown by private individuals. If you plan on harvesting this plant yourself however, just one word of caution; watch out for the thorns! Because just as the name implies this can be one prickly pear!

When this herb is commercially sold it comes with the thorns thankfully removed, but yes, if you grow them yourself you will have to remove the thorns yourself as well. Regardless of how you do it however, this one prickly little pear can do wonders to ease your weight loss.

Gurmar Leaves

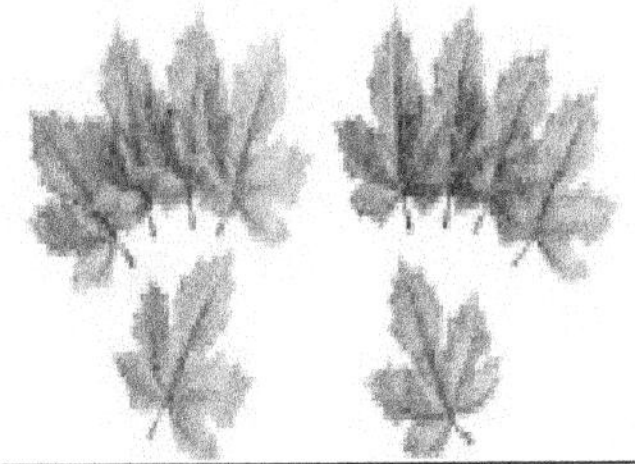

Long used as a part of Indian medicine to treat diabetes and aid in weight loss, the leaves of this plant are said to be rich in gymnemic acid that helps to curb appetite and even gets rid of sugar cravings. In fact, chewing the leaves is said to nullify sweet taste buds for up to 6 hours.

So if you have a problem reaching for sugary sweets and candies these leaves just might be a useful aid in kicking the habit. It has been used as a dietary tool of adjustment in Aruvedic circles for thousands of years. And with the name "Gurmar" which translates as "destroyer of sweetness" this herb helps to destroy the fat!

Coleus Forskohlii

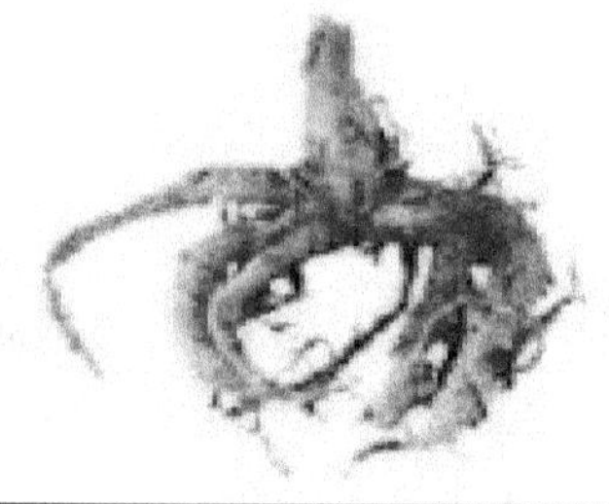

Another great herb from the mint family, the roots of this medicinal plant contains the compound from which it's name is derived; "Forskohlin". This chemical helps to regulate thyroid function, the result of this regulation is a sudden boost of energy and a curbing of your appetite.

Along with weight loss this herb has also been known to increase testosterone in men, and it is for this reason that it is mostly recommended for male consumption. It is a scientific fact that testosterone helps the body lose weight, and any supplement that increases a man's testosterone levels, whether over the counter or over the garden, will aid in this task. This root is good boiled and chopped up over salads or used in teas.

Peppermint

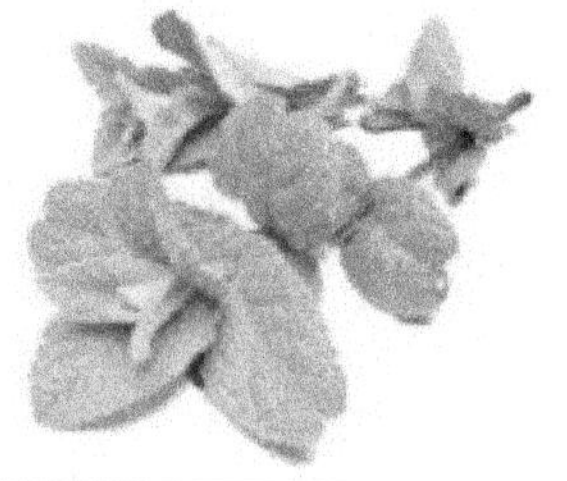

And since we are going down the list of herbs that are mints, let's finish up with the best minty weight loss herb of all; peppermint! Yes, the same plant that is responsible for those fresh tasting breath mints and your peppermint flavored beverages, is also has many powerful weight loss properties packed within its leaves.

Because besides freshening your breath, peppermint has been shown to help cleanse our system and treat digestive problems such as irritable bowl syndrome, while raising our general metabolism and putting our body in a state that is more conducive for weight loss.

Chapter 5: Herbal Remedies for a Healthy and Long Life

And now finally as we come to the last chapter in this book, we are going to take a look at the most vital aspect of any herbal routine; being able to live a longer life. Everyone is trying to live longer nowadays, and modern medicine has come a long way in aiding us.

But as we look to the future, we have to ask, are we missing something from our past? Because the ancient practice of herbal medicine has quite a bit to offer when it comes to living a healthy, happy and long life. In fact, there are quite a few stories of the herbalists of yesteryear achieving feats of longevity that would be considered impossible today.

The current expectation for a maximum human lifespan is somewhere around 120 years old. But what about a man who was rumored to have reached 197? Sounds unbelievable, but there is a long standing rumor that a man by name of Li Ching-Yun who passed away in 1933 just three years short of his 200th birthday. It may sound like a joke but many anthropologists that visited his home turf of Szechwan Province in rural China have dug up records that seem to refute the unbelievable.

And what was this mystery man's supposed secret for his long life; herbs, many, many, herbs. It was said that in one days time Li Ching-Yun would consume a vast multitude of herbs for many different reasons. No Big Mac's and Pizza for Li Ching-Yun, because his diet consisted almost completely of life enhancing medical herbs. But don't worry you don't have to devout yourself to an all herb diet, here are just a few to get you started off right!

Ginkgo Biloba

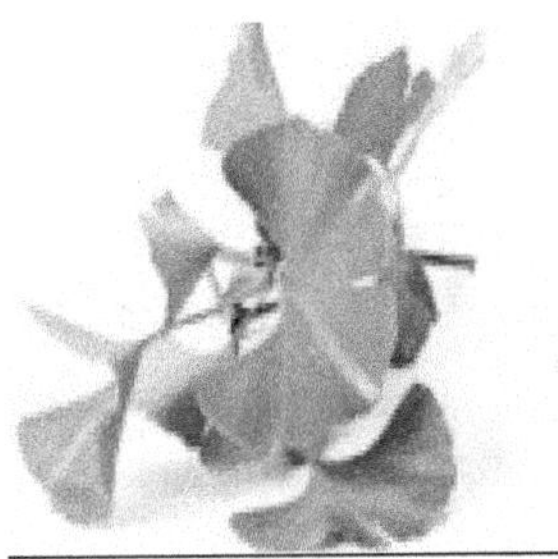

Known as the fountain of youth in China, this herb isn't far off from living up to that expectation. Even the tree from which this herb is from is known for its incredible longevity, with a life span of over 1000 years, making them among the oldest known organisms on the planet.

This herb helps to restore, shield, and protect mitochondria. This is very important if you would like to live a long time because it is the mitochondria within our cells that keep our entire body functioning properly. Healthy mitochondria are the foot soldiers of cell function and a fundamental requirement when it comes to having a long and healthy life.

Rhodiola Rosea

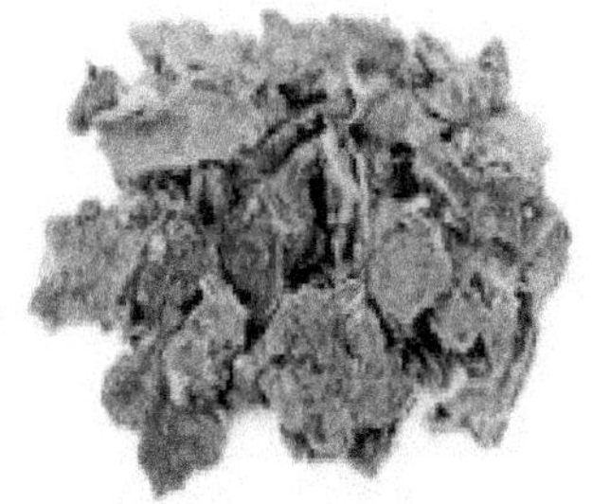

Russian researchers have spent some serious time studying this amazing herb and due to its anti-aging and healing properties it has been used by Russian Olympians and even Russian Cosmonauts. The extracts of this herb have a proven ability when it comes to repairing our DNA. This medicinal herb works directly, at the molecucle level to slow the breakdown of DNA.

And since it is the breakdown of DNA over time that causes us to age, this herb makes us live longer and better by making sure that our DNA carries on without a hitch. Along with general DNA maintenance, this herb also raises the immune system and reduces stress, adding even more benefit to all of its many other anti-aging properties.

Hawthorn

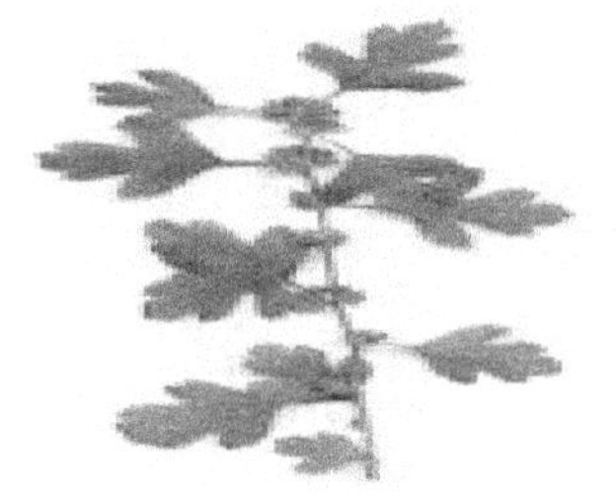

This herb is known to prolong life because of its ability to strengthen the heart. Our heart is undoubtedly the most important muscle of our body. Because needless to say, if that muscle is not doing a good enough job of pumping blood throughout our body, we are not going to live very long to complain about its poor performance.

Having a strong heart is absolutely imperative in living a long and healthy life. And for those that have suffered from heart failure, it has been discovered that adding just a little bit of Hawthorne to their diet has worked to repair and strengthen their previously damaged heart. All of these herbs promise to be great working agents for a longer and healthier life.

Conclusion: Herb your Enthusiasm!

The ancient practice of herbal remedies has been enjoying quite a revival in recent years. The enthusiasm for being able to find natural solutions to modern day health problems is greater than ever. Many studies have also been conducted to grant merit to this enthusiasm, showing that herbs can provide the same results of many over the counter prescriptions without any of the bad side effects.

Reminding us once again, that in order to truly be healthy we need to break away from our pill bottle mentality, and instead of trying to create synthetic substitutes in a lab somewhere, we should turn to nature and derive from this planet the elements that we really need to keep ourselves going strong.

I'm rather fond of the comedian Larry David who often describes people today as curbing their enthusiasm in order to impress people. But when it comes to medicinal herbs there is nothing that needs to be downplayed or toned down. So go ahead everybody and herb your enthusiasm!

FREE Bonus Reminder

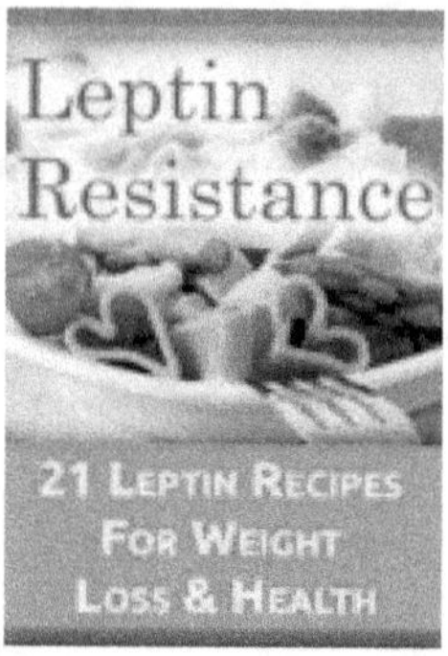

If you have not grabbed it yet, please go ahead and download your special bonus report *"Leptin Resistance. 21 Leptin Recipes For Weight Loss & Healthy Living"*.
Simply Click the Button Below

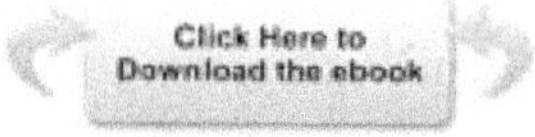

OR **Go to This Page**
http://easyweightlossway.com/free/

BONUS #2: More Free & Discounted Books

Do you want to receive more Free & Discounted Books?
We have a mailing list where we send out our new Books when they go free or with a discount on Kindle. Click on the link below to sign up for Free & Discount Book Promotions.
=> **Sign Up for Free & Discount Book Promotions** <=

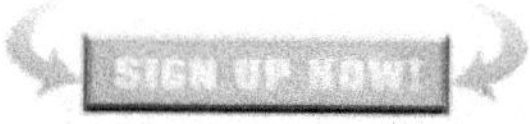

OR Go to this URL
http://zbit.ly/1WBb1Ek